Benign Anorectal Disorders - An Update

Edited by Alberto Vannelli and Daniela Cornelia Lazar

Published in London, United Kingdom

Benign Anorectal Disorders - An Update
http://dx.doi.org/10.5772/intechopen.98069
Edited by Alberto Vannelli and Daniela Cornelia Lazar

Contributors
Ignatius Riwanto, Sigit Adi Prasetyo, Parish Budiono, Damir Karlović, Dorian Kršul, Ante Jerković, Marko Zelić, Đordano Bačić, Bengi Balci, Sezai Leventoglu, Bulent Mentes, Esther María Cano Pecharromán, A. Teresa Calderón Duque, Juan Carlos Santiago Peña, Tomás Balsa Marín, Nikolaos Andromanakos, Dimitrios Filippou, Alkiviadis Kostakis, Alana Padilha Fontanella, Léo Dantas Pereira, Maria Julia Segantini, Omar Féres, Sthefânia Frizol, Rafael Luis Luporini, Nathalie Mantilla, Juaquito Jorge, Octavio Gómez-Escudero, René Dembélé, Wendpoulomdé A.D. Kaboré, Issiaka Soulama, Oumar Traoré, Nafissatou Ouédraogo, Ali Konaté, Nathalie K. Guessennd, David Coulibaly N'Golo, Antoine Sanou, Samuel Serme, Soumanaba Zongo, Emmanuel Sampo, Alfred S. Traoré, Amy Gassama-Sow, Nicholas Barro, Muhammad Asrar, Zeeshan Javed, Bilal Rasool, Rabia Batool, Mohammad Asad Mangat, Usama Saleem, Muhammad Imran, Amna Batool, Daniela Cornelia Lazar, Elena-Alina Moacă, Mărioara Cornianu, Sorina Tăban, Alexandra Faur, Adrian Goldiş

First published in London, United Kingdom, 2023 by IntechOpen
IntechOpen is the global imprint of INTECHOPEN LIMITED, registered in England and Wales, registration number: 11086078, 5 Princes Gate Court, London, SW7 2QJ, United Kingdom

British Library Cataloguing-in-Publication Data
A catalogue record for this book is available from the British Library

Additional hard and PDF copies can be obtained from orders@intechopen.com

Benign Anorectal Disorders - An Update
Edited by Alberto Vannelli and Daniela Cornelia Lazar
p. cm.
Print ISBN 978-1-80355-705-2
Online ISBN 978-1-80355-706-9
eBook (PDF) ISBN 978-1-80355-707-6

For EU product safety concerns:
IN TECH d.o.o., Prolaz Marije Krucifikse Kozulić 3, 51000 Rijeka, Croatia,
info@intechopen.com or visit our website at intechopen.com.

Meet the editors

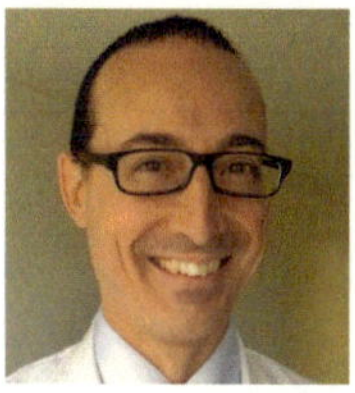

Alberto Vannelli attended medical school and completed post-graduate research and general surgical training in Milan before training in colorectal surgery at the National Cancer Institute and eventually joining the faculty there. Over the 10 years that followed, he played an instrumental role in developing what was widely considered the finest department of colorectal surgery in the world. He is currently director of general surgery at Valduce Hospital, Como, Italy, a referral center for a colorectal disease that is known for sphincter-saving procedures for rectal cancer and for treatment of inflammatory bowel disease (IBD). Dr. Vannelli focuses on advanced minimally invasive techniques, including multidisciplinary management of patients with colorectal cancers. He has participated as a speaker at national and international meetings and has published several publications in peer-reviewed journals. In 2012, Dr. Vannelli founded Erone Onlus to assist cancer patients and their families. He collaborates with the School of Specialization in General Surgery at the Emergency Department of the University of Milan.

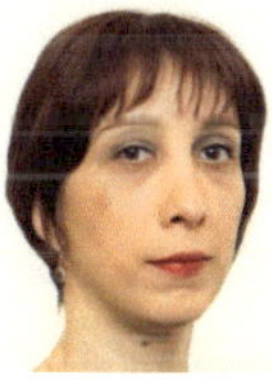

Dr. Daniela Lazar is an associate professor in the Department of Internal Medicine at the University of Medicine and Pharmacy Timișoara, Romania. She began her career in the Department of Gastroenterology and Hepatology at the same university, where she acquired clinical skills in gastroenterology, learned the techniques of endoscopy and abdominal ultrasonography and began her research activity. She is specialized in Gastroenterology, Internal Medicine and Medical Oncology and underwent completed her Ph.D. thesis in the field of gastric cancer. Dr. Lazar's research interests are concerned mainly with the neoplasms of the gastrointestinal tract, especially gastric cancer. She has published many studies regarding angiogenesis, premalignant lesions, prognostic factors and novel therapies in gastric cancer in prestigious journals, with numerous citations. She is a reviewer for many international journals. She is also interested in aspects of the epidemiology, phenotypes, and treatment of inflammatory bowel disease and is a member of national and international working groups in this domain. Dr. Lazar has taken part in many national and international congresses with research studies in the field of gastroenterology and digestive oncology.

Contents

Preface

Benign anorectal disorders carry significant morbidity and financial burdens for the healthcare system. Benign anorectal disorders of structure and function are common in clinical practice. A patient consulting a doctor with anorectal complaints is likely to have progressed to the point of extreme discomfort.

Understanding anorectal anatomy is key to evaluating patients with the benign anorectal disease. The anorectal area is the terminal portion of the lower gastrointestinal tract. It is a part of the pelvic district that includes the urogenital organs and muscular, ligamentous, and connective tissue structures. As a functional unit, the anorectal area maintains fecal continence by acting as both a reservoir and an expulsion unit for feces.

The rectum has both intraperitoneal and extraperitoneal segments. The rectum begins at the confluence of the taeniae coli at the rectosigmoid junction. We commonly define the rectum as the last 12 cm above the anal verge. The anal canal is roughly 4 cm in length and extends from the anal verge to the proximal level of the levator – the external anal sphincter complex. The sphincter mechanisms and the dentate line are of great importance when addressing the anal canal surgically.

The dentate line (pectinate line) is approximately 2 cm from the anal verge and is a place of transition from columnar epithelium (endoderm) to squamous epithelium (ectoderm). Between these layers is a transitional area called the cloacogenic zone. The dentate line divides the upper two-thirds from the lower third of the anal canal. Developmentally, this line represents the hindgut proctodeum junction, an important landmark because of differences in innervation, blood supply, and lymphatic drainage of the anal canal; several distinctions and pathologies are based upon the location of a structure relative to this line. The anal glands, of which there are typically four to eight, empty into the anal canal at the base of the anal columns. These extend through the full thickness of the mucosa and submucosa and even into the muscularis externa. They are branched, straight tubular glands with ducts lined with stratified columnar epithelium, and their function is mucus secretion.

For any problem, performing taking a complete history and performing a physical examination is mandatory. Bleeding, pain, discharge, swelling, changes in bowel habits, pruritus, prolapse, fever, incontinence, prior sexual contacts, and dyspareunia, are valuable information. Digital rectal and bimanual examinations are mandatory. Also important are sphincter tone, presence of gross blood, and presence or absence of hemorrhoids. Endoscopy (ano- and proctoscopy) is among the possible diagnostic tests. During the physical examination, temperature, body habitus, the abdomen, and the perineum require special attention.

This book summarizes the preferred approach to the evaluation and management of defecation disorders, proctalgia syndromes, hemorrhoids, anal fissures, and fecal incontinence in adults. Each section contains key concepts, recommendations, and summaries of the available evidence. Written by highly experienced physicians, the book provides detailed notes on the optimal management of these disorders including pre-and post-operative management. The chapters cover the entire range of benign disorders such as hemorrhoids, fissures, fistula-in-ano, anorectal injuries, anal incontinence, rectal prolapse, pelvic floor disorders, benign tumors and ulcers, and strictures.

Alberto Vannelli
Director,
General Surgery,
Valduce Hospital,
Como, Italy

Daniela Cornelia Lazar
Victor Babeș University of Medicine and Pharmacy,
Timișoara, Romania

Section 1

Anal Fistula

Chapter 1

Anal Fistula: Contemporary View of Complex Problem

Damir Karlović, Dorian Kršul, Ante Jerković, Đordano Bačić and Marko Zelić

Abstract

Anal fistulas are still a huge challenge for surgeons because of their high incidence, high recurrence rate, prolonged healing time and possible complications such as fecal incontinence. Even though many surgical options have been described, we still do not have the standardized procedure. Patients who suffered from this problem have a low quality of life because of constant anal pain and soiling from anal tracts. Aside from cryptoglandular etiology, fistulas associated with Crohn's disease are separate entity that requires a multidisciplinary approach. This chapter will be an overview of modern approaches in anal fistula treatment regardless of etiology with special consideration on how to avoid adverse outcomes and to improve patients' quality of life.

Keywords: anal fistula, fecal incontinence, cryptoglandular, IBD, sphincter preserving techniques

1. Introduction

Anal fistulas, especially complex anal fistulas, still present a challenge for surgeons because of their high recurrence rate, possible postoperative risk of fecal incontinence and also the fact that nowadays we still do not have a standardized procedure of choice for treatment.

An anal fistula is defined as an abnormal communication between perianal skin and anal canal, filled with granulation and fibrotic tissue that supports chronic inflammation, disabling spontaneous healing. Most fistulas are of cryptoglandular etiology, but can also be associated with inflammatory bowel disease (Mb Crohn), malignancies, trauma, pelvic sepsis or diverticulitis. Incidence of the disease is about 10 cases per 100,000 individuals with a male to female ratio of 2:1 [1, 2].

In the past, various classifications for anal fistulas were proposed. One of the most widespread classifications was Parks' classification which classified fistulas according to their correlation with anal sphincter complex and divided fistulas into intersphincteric, transsphincteric, suprasphincteric and extrasphincteric [3].

Surgeons noticed, using traditional surgical techniques such as fistulotomy, fistulectomy or cutting seton, frequent continence disturbance following operations, especially in cases when fistula tract passed through deeper parts of sphincter complex and internal fistula opening was positioned more proximally in the anal canal.

To simplify classification and to prevent possible postoperative continence disturbance, colorectal surgeons nowadays mostly use simple classification which divides fistulas into two groups: simple and complex, according to the relation of the proportion of the anal sphincter mechanism they pass through. The classification that distinguishes simple and complex anal fistulas helps the surgeon to avoid using traditional techniques to prevent possible continence disturbance, but does not help in the decision which operative technique is best to use in the treatment of complex fistulas. Classification by Garg is extrapolated from multiple clinical scenarios and presents a better correlation with an actual patient case (**Figure 1**).

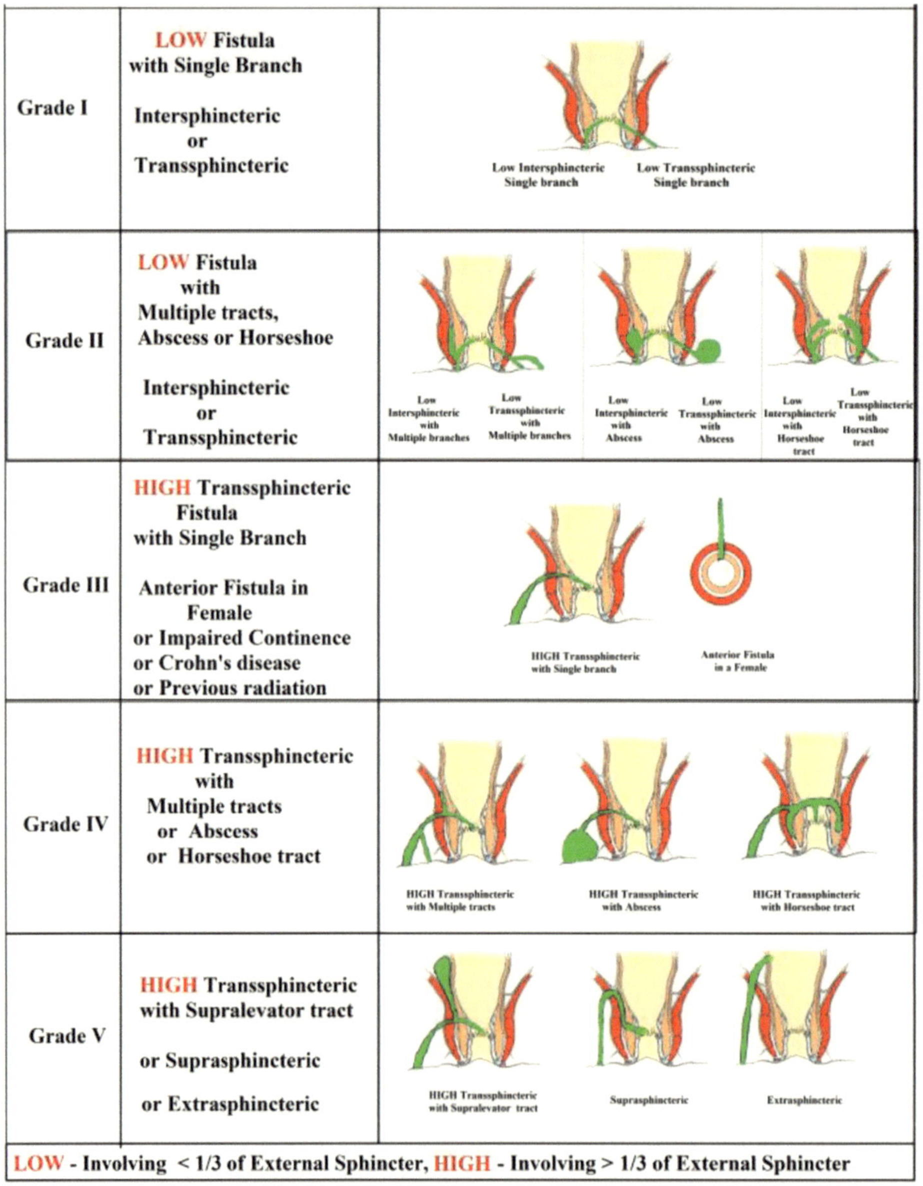

Figure 1.
Garg classification of anal fistulas (with permission of Dr. Pankaj Garg).

Simple anal fistulas have only one tract that crosses less than 30% of the anal sphincter complex and can be treated by fistulotomy or fistulectomy with very low postoperative continence disturbance incidence and high healing rate.

All other fistulas are classified as complex. These fistulas cross the anal sphincter at a point that encompasses more than 30% of the external anal sphincter. They can have multiple tracts. Complex fistulas also include those about inflamatory bowel disease (IBD), those which are anteriorly positioned in female patients or those which are recurrent. If those fistulas are treated with fistulotomy or some other traditional technique, it can result in some type of postoperative fecal incontinence. The average rate of continence disturbance, such as flatus or liquid stool leakage following fistulotomy, was observed in 20–25% cases and up to 12% cases after cutting seton treatment [4, 5]. This effect on continence has resulted in traditional surgical techniques being less favorable for complex anal fistulas treatment and the incentive to use minimally invasive sphincter sparing techniques is increasing.

In anal fistula treatment, it is important to apply an appropriate surgical approach to obtain the best postoperative results such as high primary healing rate, low postoperative pain, low risk for any type of fecal incontinence, low recurrence rate and to subsequently increase postoperative patient's life quality.

2. Goals of anal fistula treatment

2.1 Pathogenesis

To delve into the intricacies of anal fistulas, one must first understand hypotheses that currently exist. The most widespread hypothesis is the cryptoglandular one which states that infected or inflamed anal glands are the cause of anal abscess and fistula [6]. This could be due to the ascending inflammation originating in the anal canal or blockage of discharge. Over almost 150 years, much research was done to find out exact relationship between anal glands and anal fistula, and while some researchers found them to correlate, others weren't even able to prove the existence of anal glands or found them to be very variable at best [7]. Nevertheless, this is the predominant theory that surgeons adhere to throughout the modern surgery era, and anal glands seem to be the likely culprit. Despite this, etiology remains uncertain or unknown, but the inflammatory process seems to play a crucial role.

From the anatomical standpoint, it was stated by Parks that anal fistula is the chronic manifestation of anal abscess that is an acute condition. Fistula forms as a consequence of the medio-lateral spread of infection that subsequently may perforate the anal sphincter complex and extend to the perianal skin, thus forming a fistula [3]. More recently, Garg has shown that intersphincteric space plays a major role in anal fistula pathology, stating that almost all complex fistulas have some degree of intersphincteric involvement and that fistula in closed intersphincteric space acts like an abscess and must be treated accordingly [8, 9].

Molecular analyses of an anal fistula are scarce. One study has shown abundant expression of pro-inflammatory cytokine IL-1b in 93 % of the cryptoglandular anal fistulas, along with increased levels of cytokines IL-8, IL-12p40 and TNF-α in anal fistulas [10]. IL-1, especially IL-1β are strong pro-inflammatory cytokines that can be stimulated by other cytokines, microbial products and even IL-1β by auto stimulation, which can play a role in the recurrence or persistence of anal fistula. Tozer et al. showed immunological differences between cryptoglandular and Crohn's disease-associated fistula [11]. While those are undoubtedly valuable findings that advance our understanding of anal fistula pathology, they still don't change anything in our management of this problem.

2.2 Diagnostic methods for anal fistulas

To achieve best results, accomplish a higher primary healing rate, prevent recurrence and risk of postoperative continence disturbance, it is essential to identify the entire course of fistula tract including infected anal gland in intersphincteric space, main and possible secondary tracts. In that way, one can decide which surgical option is best for the patient.

After performing DRE, additional usage of the metal probe with insertion through fistula canal should be done to identify which type of fistula patient has so one can decide which surgical option should be performed. In case of pain, this can be performed under anesthesia (EUA: examination under anesthesia) [12]. In the case of a simple anal fistula, it is usually sufficient to examine as mentioned above, but in cases of a complex anal fistula in most cases, additional diagnostic methods should be done.

Some diagnostic methods that have previously been used to verify the course of fistula tracts, have since been abandoned. One of these techniques is X-ray fistulography. This technique is not performed anymore because it does not show the correlation of the fistula tract to the anal sphincter complex, so in that way, surgeon does not know which type of anal fistula the patient has [13].

Possible options to verify the correlation of the fistula tract with anal sphincter complex are: CT fistulography, endoanal ultrasound (EUS) and MRI fistulography.

CT fistulography can be more accurate in cases associated with acute inflammations and abscesses, but it somewhat deficient in cases of mature anal fistula.

Endoanal ultrasound (EUS) is a very good option to verify fistula tract correlation with sphincter complex and possible secondary branches but it is a highly operator-dependent technique [14–16].

For now, the golden standard for anal fistula diagnosis and classification is magnetic resonance imaging (MRI). MRI helps not only to accurately demonstrate disease extension but also to predict prognosis, make therapy decisions and can be used in some cases in follow-up periods especially in the patient suffering from Crohn´s disease or recurrent fistula (**Figure 2**) [16–21].

One other possibility in the verification of main fistula tract and possible secondary branches is using fistuloscope during the diagnostic phase of VAAFT procedure (video-assisted anal fistula treatment) but the technique can also be considered as operator-dependent [22]. VAAFT procedure will be discussed later in this chapter.

2.3 Management principles

It is stated that the ideal treatment for anal fistula lies on two principles. The first is the eradication of sepsis and promotion of fistula tract healing, and the second is preserving the sphincter complex and continence mechanism [23]. With simple fistulas, this can be achieved by laying open the fistulous tract with high healing rates and with no significant continence disturbance [24]. While simple fistulas have simple treatment solutions, the concept of treatment for complex fistulas is somewhat different, and while the above-mentioned principle holds, certain aspects should be explained.

Colorectal surgeons' postulate that internal fistula openings should always be identified and closed. This was shown in a meta-analysis by Mei et al. with class I

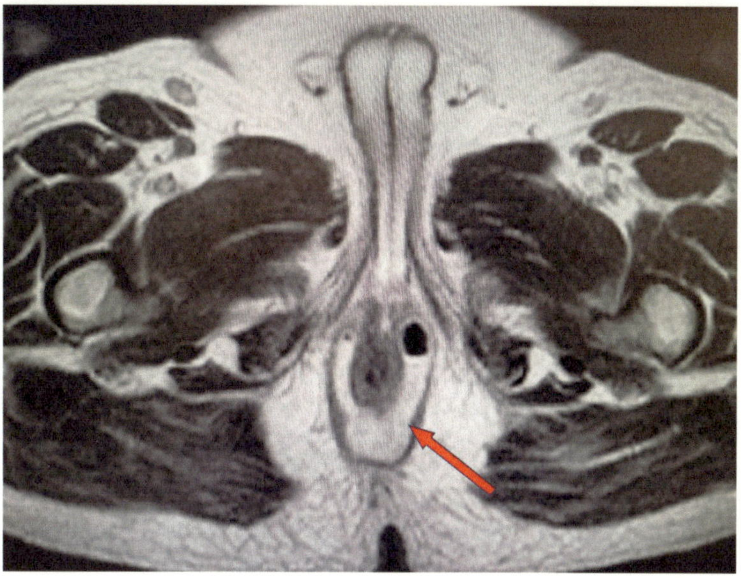

Figure 2.
MR fistulography clearly shows horseshoe fistula on axial view.

evidence for significant association between anal fistula recurrence and failure to identify and close internal fistula opening. The same meta-analysis also showed the connection between horseshoe fistula extensions and recurrence [25]. Both of these problems could be solved by applying video-assisted approach in treatment. This covers the first principle.

To achieve the second principle in complex anal fistula, sphincter preserving techniques should be used to address the anal continence problem. Currently, no study compares lay open techniques and sphincter preserving techniques for complex anal fistula treatment but other studies have shown that, in this case, lay open techniques have an unacceptably high incidence of continence disturbance, up to 25% [4]. Meanwhile, sphincter preserving techniques for complex fistulas, with the possible exception of rectal advancement flap, have shown to have no or only minor continence disturbances in up to 1.7% patients [26].

A somewhat different approach, arising from analysis of modern sphincter preserving techniques, to the ideal treatment of anal fistulas was described by Garg. He hypothesized that in order to successfully heal anal fistula, we should bear in mind three principles:

1. Intersphincteric fistula tract acts like an abscess in closed intersphincteric space.

2. Second principle follows the first: intersphincteric fistula must be drained and continuous drainage should be ensured.

3. Healing occurs progressively until interrupted irreversibly by a collection [9].

This may be the reason why most sphincter preserving treatment methods still do not have healing results comparable to lay open techniques.

3. Traditional surgical techniques: fistulotomy, fistulectomy, seton placement

When talking about traditional techniques in anal fistula treatment we refer to fistulotomy, fistulectomy or techniques with seton placement in the anal fistula canal. Even since Hippocrates, there have been advices and different references on how one should treat anal fistula [27]. Traditional techniques were used in the treatment of anal fistula during history, before the development of sphincter preserving techniques.

Fistulotomy as the oldest, simplest and most widely performed procedure in anal fistula treatment has its benefits and drawbacks. This procedure, with its synonym "lay open technique," is quite a simple procedure in which the surgeon, after insertion of the metal probe, cuts (or lays open) the whole of fistula tract from the internal fistula opening which is located in the anal canal to the external opening situated on the perianal skin. Following this, the surgeon performs curettement of granulation tissue from the fistula tract remnant making, in a sense, an acute wound that should heal by secondary intention. Some surgeons perform additional marsupialization of wound edges the following fistulotomy to reduce postoperative bleeding and to speed up wound healing (**Figure 3**) [28].

In this way, crucial postulates in anal fistula treatment are satisfied, except the preservation of anal sphincter complex to a lesser degree. Even though this procedure has a success rate of more than 90%, it is also associated with some type of postoperative continence disturbance in cases when the fistula tract crosses through deeper parts of the anal sphincter complex and when the internal fistula opening is placed more proximally in the anal canal. The incontinence rate following these procedures vary given the heterogeneity of anal fistulas, but can be up to 28% [4, 29].

In recent times, according to Garg's classification, this technique should be only reserved for treatment of type 1 and 2 anal fistulae without risk of continence disturbance, meaning low intersphincteric and low transsphincteric fistula (simple anal fistula) [30].

Fistulectomy is performed by excising the whole of fistula tract, removing in that way the whole fistula tract from external fistula opening to internal fistula opening, without preservation of anal sphincter complex. In a meta-analysis that included

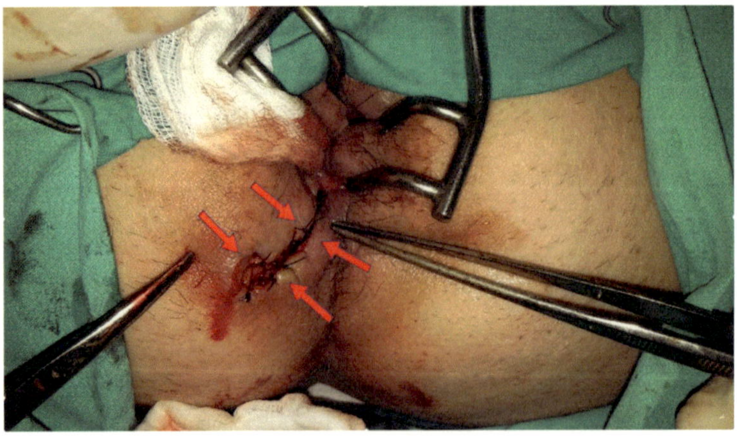

Figure 3.
Fistulotomy with marsupialization (shown by red arrows).

565 patients comparing fistulectomy and fistulotomy for low anal fistulas, there has been no conclusive evidence as to which procedure is better in simple anal fistula treatment [31].

Failure of treatment with fistulotomy of fistulectomy and recurrence is associated with inappropriate selection of patients with high anal fistulas or those with multiple tracts.

The seton placement technique distinguishes between "cutting" and "loose" seton.

Cutting seton technique is nowadays almost abandoned but was used to convert high anal fistula to low one which was later treated by lay open technique. Seton was made of unabsorbable material, placed through the anal fistula canal and then tightened enabling in that way slow cutting of the sphincter mechanism leaving behind a scar. The idea behind the technique was that it would prevent anal sphincter muscle to split and, in that way, to prevent serious problems with continence disturbance. It was proven however, that this technique has a high incidence of continence disturbance with high morbidity and recurrence rates [5].

When talking about the role of loose seton the situation is somewhat different. Loose seton should be placed through the fistula tract without tightening, helping in that way to reduce sepsis and to mature the fistula tract. This would be the first stage in resolving of anal fistula problem. Many surgeons advocate loose seton placement as an important step of rectal advancement flap procedure or LIFT (ligation of intersphincteric fistula tract) prior to that operation, even though there has not been clear clinical evidence [32, 33]. Seton placement before fistulotomy with sphincter reconstruction has shown its benefits in fistula treatment, namely in converting high transsphincteric to low transsphincteric fistula and also in the acute abscess stage before this procedure to reduce the risk of breakdown of sphincter repair [34].

4. Sphincter preserving techniques: new solutions to prevent postoperative fecal incontinence

As mentioned earlier, the high risk of postoperative continence disturbance after treatment of complex anal fistulas with traditional techniques, have led to the need for the development of new techniques, which would be dubbed "sphincter preserving techniques." The main characteristic of such techniques is that they prevent or greatly reduce any possibility of postoperative fecal incontinence. Various sphincter preserving techniques were introduced in clinical practice in the last 10–15 years. Among these are laser treatment procedure (FiLaC®: fistula laser closure), fibrin glue treatment, anal fistula plug, VAAFT procedure (video-assisted anal fistula treatment), LIFT procedure (ligation of intersphincteric fistula tract), anal fistula treatment with platelet cells (PRP: platelet rich plasma), RAF (rectal advancement flap) and others [22, 33, 35–42].

Some sphincter preserving techniques weren't broadly accepted given high cost, high recurrence rates or inability to reproduce similar results in other centers. Of above-mentioned sphincter preserving techniques, several gained wider acceptance, such as LIFT, VAAFT, and RAF technique.

4.1 Ligation of intersphincteric fistula tract (LIFT)

Ligation of intersphincteric fistula tract (LIFT) is a sphincter preserving technique first performed and published by Rojanasakul [39]. This technique satisfies all goals of anal fistula treatment such as the closure of internal fistula opening, removal of infected intersphincteric fistula tract (anal gland) and eradication of remaining fistula tract. It is reserved for the treatment of complex transsphincteric anal fistulas. After identification of fistula tract using metal, probe surgeon makes a curvilinear incision on the anocutaneous border entering intersphincteric space and performs preparation of intersphincteric part of anal fistula, followed by removal of the intersphincteric portion of the fistula. Closure of remaining defect of anal fistula on internal and external anal sphincter muscle then follows. Curettement of remaining fistula tract from external fistula opening to external anal sphincter muscle should be performed. Intersphincteric space is then reconstructed and the perianal wound sutured.

According to the two available meta-analyses, this procedure gives an overall success rate of 76.4 and 78 % respectively, with a low complication rate 5.5–13.9%. The most common complication was wound dehiscence, and others were bleeding, infection, hematoma, anal discharge. Only a low grade of postoperative fecal incontinence in 1.4% of patents was recorded (**Figure 4**) [33, 43].

This technique is easily reproducible without the necessity of investment in potentially expensive equipment. In case of dehiscence of intersphincteric space loose seton can be inserted through the intersphincteric wound, thus making conversion of transsphincteric fistula in intersphincteric one, which can be afterward treated by fistulotomy without fear of continence disturbance.

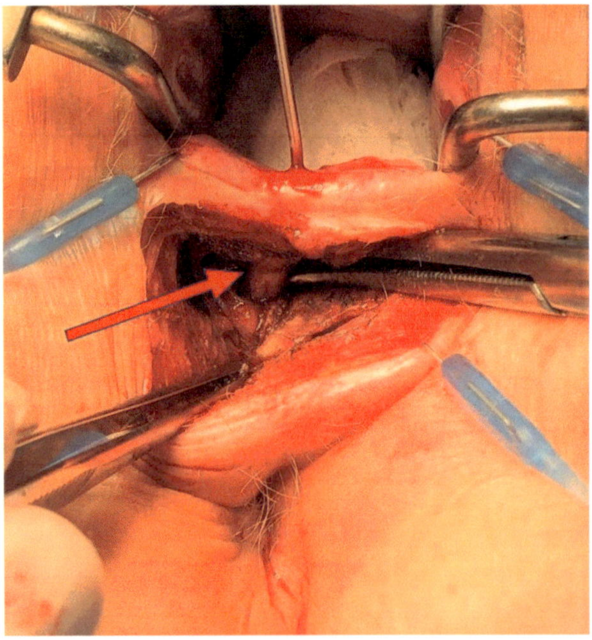

Figure 4.
LIFT procedure: identification of fistula tract in the intersphincteric plane; red arrow showing fistula tract.

4.2 Video-assisted anal fistula treatment (VAAFT)

Video-assisted anal fistula treatment (VAAFT) procedure is the only technique that enables visualization and operation of anal fistula from within fistula tract, using specially designed equipment. This sphincter preserving technique was developed by Meinero who described short and long-term results [22].

Using a special instrument (fistuloscope), the surgeon visualizes the fistula tract from inside, which helps to identify possible secondary branches of the fistula tract,

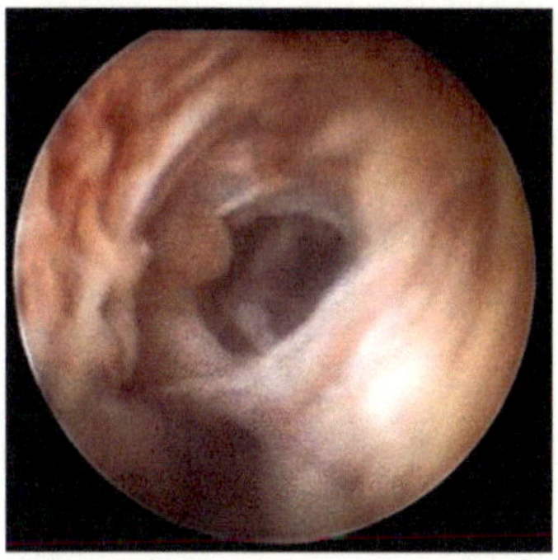

Figure 5.
Intraoperative view of the fistula tract through fistuloscope.

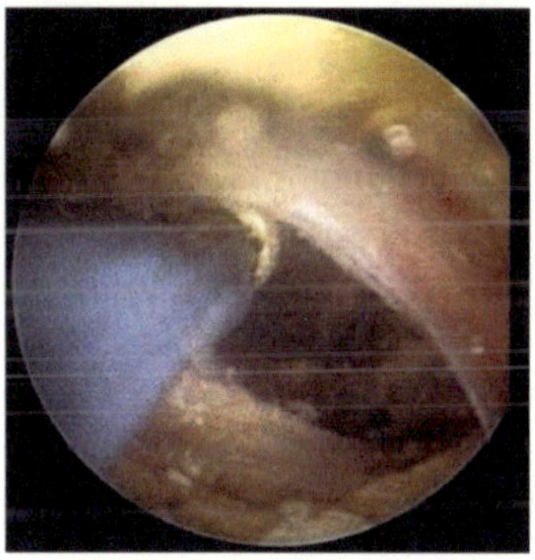

Figure 6.
Fulguration of the fistulous tract.

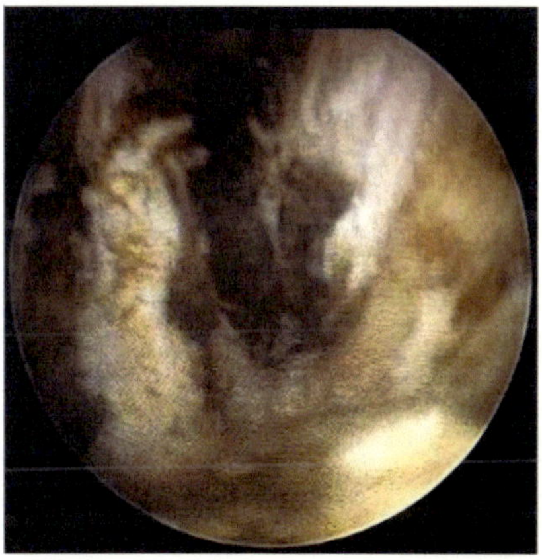

Figure 7.
View of the debris after fulguration.

abscess cavities and later destroys all chronic granulation tissue in the fistula tract making in that way an acute wound which should heal by secondary intention. The important part of this technique is also to identify the internal fistula opening inside the anal canal and to close it securely (**Figures 5–9**).

Many surgeons worldwide accepted this technique in their everyday practice for the treatment of complex anal fistulas [22, 38, 44–46].

The main indication for this technique is the treatment of complex anal fistulas, especially cases with multiple secondary branches which are deep in

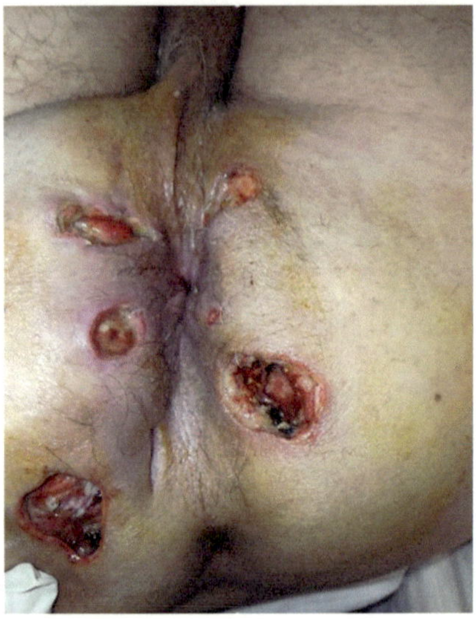

Figure 8.
Postoperative view after VAAFT for complex horseshoe fistula.

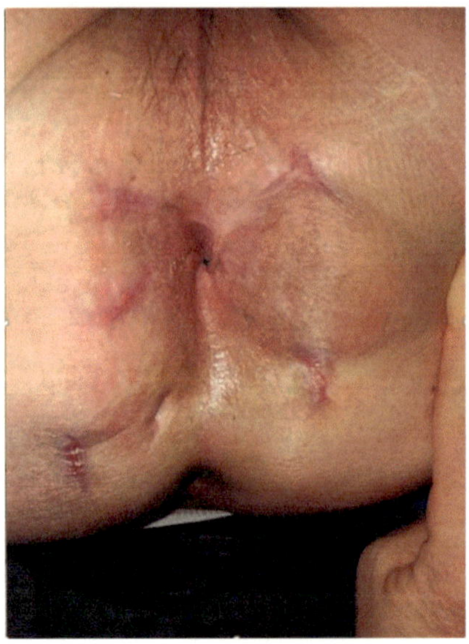

Figure 9.
Healed wounds in the same patient.

the ischioanal fossa and are not easily reached. Also, VAAFT has its benefits in treatment of patients who have anal fistula associated with Crohn's disease, helping to ameliorate symptoms associated with chronic anal fistula such as pain and soiling, thus significantly increasing patient's quality of life [44, 47]. VAAFT technique is comparable with other sphincter preserving techniques to healing and patient satisfaction. Diminished postoperative pain, earlier recovery after surgery and smaller postoperative perianal wounds allows for earlier return to normal activities [48].

In case of failure, this technique can be repeated because there is no risk for any continence disturbance following this procedure. The proposed mechanism whereby repeated procedures have an incremental effect is the conversion of complex fistula with multiple tracts into a more manageable, low or simple fistula, which can be called conversion of the fistula [38].

VAAFT technique has been proven to be a safe procedure, associated with good functional outcomes and a very low incidence of complications [22, 44, 45], which was shown in a published meta-analysis [46]. It showed a recurrence rate ranging from 7.5 to 33.3% with a weighted mean recurrence rate of 17.7%. Recurrence rates varied significantly depending on the method of internal fistula opening closure (mattress suture, stapler, rectal advancement flap). No affection of anal continence was documented.

4.3 Rectal advancement flap (RAF)

This technique is one of the oldest techniques which were and still are reserved for the treatment of complex anal fistulas especially in cases with large internal fistula opening. When discussing this technique, we can't talk about the "pure" sphincter preserving technique because flap should be performed by dissection of anorectal mucosa and adjacent internal anal sphincter muscle, so in that way, internal anal sphincter muscle does not stay intact.

When doing this procedure surgeon should identify and excise the internal fistula opening in the anal canal. Then the U-shaped or rhomboid flap with a wider base side should be performed by dissecting anorectal mucosa and adjacent internal anal sphincter muscle. Curettement and irrigation of the whole fistula tract should be performed, followed by suture of a defect in sphincter complex left by earlier fistula tract. The site is then a covered by previously prepared flap and sutured. Even though much research has been made about optimal flap thickness, researchers found that there was a statistically higher rate of primary healing in cases with thicker flaps, but also have noticed a higher rate of mild postoperative continence disturbance which was more severe than the thicker flap was (**Figure 10**) [41, 49, 50].

There have been many publications and several systematic reviews and meta-analyses on this technique where the effectiveness was shown to be 60–80%, but the same cases also reported some degree of postoperative fecal disturbance [42, 50, 51].

Factors that could affect healing after flap procedure are obesity and smoking, so patients should be advised to quit smoking and to try to reduce their weight prior to flap operation [52–54]. To increase the effectiveness of this technique one should perform bigger rhomboid or U-shape flaps using the minimally invasive approach, avoiding tissue trauma made by surgical cautery, avoiding excessive grasping as well as the too big strain of suture line.

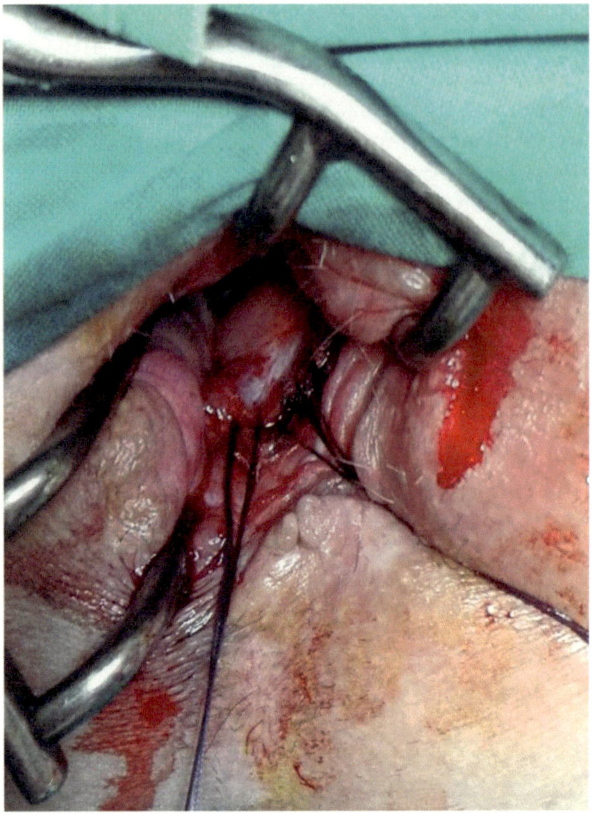

Figure 10.
Formed rectal advancement flap.

5. Other solutions for anal fistula treatment

As mentioned earlier in this chapter, there is no universal approach for anal fistula treatment. Some other possible solutions may be hybrid sphincter preserving techniques, fistulotomy with primary sphincter reconstruction, TROPIS (trans anal opening of the intersphincteric space) and use of autologous platelet rich plasma in anal fistula treatment.

5.1 Hybrid sphincter preserving techniques

Hybrid sphincter preserving techniques are combinations of two or more sphincter preserving techniques in a single procedure to increase healing rates and achieving better results.

Several reports exist with different combinations of techniques with authors trying to achieve higher healing rates, but the majority of reports are on a single institution basis or case reports with a small number of patients.

A combination of VAAFT and LIFT techniques was performed with intention of secure closure of internal fistula opening from intersphincteric space and additional exploration and eradication of remaining fistula tract from external fistula opening with identification of possible secondary branches using fistuloscope [55, 56]. VAAFT was also used in different combinations with other sphincter preserving techniques such as FiLaC® procedure and with RAF procedure in cases with large internal fistula opening [38, 44, 57].

The combination of LIFT technique with the insertion of a bioprosthetic graft in intersphincteric space was also described in a study that included 31 patients, where the success rate was 94% in a one-year follow-up period [58]. Another study combined LIFT and human acellular dermal matrix as a bioprosthetic plug with a reported success rate of 95% on a 21-patient sample [59]. Rectal advancement flap with the injection of porcine dermal collagen implant through the external opening was combined in a study which included 24 patients with a success rate of 82.5% in a 14-month follow-up period [60].

It was to be expected that surgeons started to combine two or more sphincter preserving techniques to achieve better results, but until evidence is found that one technique, or combination of techniques, has significantly better results over the others, they should be tailored individually depending on patient's case.

5.2 Fistulotomy with primary sphincter reconstruction

This approach in the treatment of anal fistulas has the same operative philosophy as fistulotomy or fistulectomy, but is reserved for higher fistulas. In this procedure surgeon after eradication of the fistula tract and possible secondary fistula branches to prevent recurrences, makes additional anal sphincter reconstruction to try to eliminate the possibility of postoperative fecal incontinence. Ratto et al. reported a 93.2% overall success rate with a low morbidity rate using this approach. Overall postoperative fecal incontinence was 12.4% mainly post-defecation soiling, without significant changes in anorectal manometry parameters [61]. Voon et al. reported their experience in using this technique and had good outcomes with a very low rate of continence disturbance in follow-up period [34]. Even though this technique has been implemented in guidelines for anal fistula treatment by several surgical societies, it wasn't accepted worldwide as the standardized procedure [62]. In case of abscess formation as the initial presentation, it is crucial to place seton drainage to give enough time for maturing of the fistula and to prevent continence disturbance following fistulotomy.

5.3 Trans anal opening of the intersphincteric space (TROPIS)

This technique was described and published by Garg, who used this approach in the treatment of high complex anal fistulas with a high primary healing rate and very low incidence of morbidities [8]. It is well known that high intersphincteric parts of anal fistula and abscesses are difficult to reach through intersphincteric approach or probing from external fistula opening, as well as that they are usually branching.

TROPIS approach also satisfies golden principles in the treatment of anal fistula such as identification and resolving internal fistula opening problem, as well as intersphincteric fistula tract with the accompanying anal gland, and also eradication of remaining fistulous tract by curettement.

The procedure is done by laying open intersphincteric space through internal anal with preservation of external sphincter. The external tracts in the ischioanal fossa should be curetted and the intersphincteric space is left open for secondary healing. In the initial prospective cohort which included 61 patients, the success rate was 84.6%

with no significant changes with continence. The study included patients with high transsphincteric (anterior and posterior) and high intersphincteric type of fistula [8].

TROPIS procedure is an excellent approach for posterior high transsphincteric type and high intersphincteric type of anal fistula, especially if transsphincteric fistula is located at the puborectalis level. However, combination with drainage (preoperative seton placement and postoperative drain placement in remaining tract from external fistula opening), curettement or excision of external tracts is necessary to reduce recurrences.

5.4 Use of autologous platelet rich plasma in anal fistula treatment

Autologous platelet rich plasma (APRP) is nowadays used in various fields of medicine such as orthopedics, plastic surgery, dental medicine, but also in the treatment of anal fistula in the last decade. APRP is platelet concentration derived from centrifuged full blood after removal of red blood cells. Such prepared plasma is a rich source of various growth factors implicated in regeneration and tissue healing [63, 64].

The procedure consists of curettement of fistula tract and closure of internal fistula opening with an additional injection of previously prepared platelet rich autologous blood sample [65]. The majority of publications combined mucosal advancement flap with APRP injection [65–67]. Several publications reported an average healing rate from 60 to 90% [40, 66–68]. The drawbacks of mentioned publications were that they had a relatively small number of patients enrolled and still no meta-analyses exist on the subject. No problem with any type of postoperative fecal incontinence was reported. This is still considered to be a somewhat experimental procedure and is not widely used. The platelet separation procedure requires special equipment that is often only available in larger institutions. Also cost per patient exceeds that of the other techniques, which is why this technique needs more solid evidence for a patient benefit before it can be considered to become one of the mainstream sphincters preserving treatments.

6. Anal fistula in Crohn's disease

We can say that fistulas associated with Crohn's disease present a special entity in the treatment of anal fistulas. This kind of fistula presents a huge challenge for surgeons despite numerous surgical possibilities and technical advancements in recent years. Symptoms associated with Crohn's anal fistula include purulent drainage, severe pain, possible continence disturbance which all can lead to a significant reduction in quality of life. These kinds of fistulas are often recurrent and hard to treat. The incidence of anal fistulas in patients with Crohn's disease is 5 to 40% and is more common in patients who have a higher severity of colorectal inflammation [69–71].

Even though numerous surgical techniques have been described for the treatment of this kind of anal fistulas, the choice of which technique is best often depends on the anatomy, presence of local inflammation, type of fistula, and surgeon's experience (**Figure 11**) [72–74].

Many management proposals have been published, but all had higher reports of postoperative complications such as continence disturbance, infection and high recurrence rate compared to the same type of fistulas not associated with Crohn's disease. Currently, numerous novel surgical sphincters preserving techniques are being

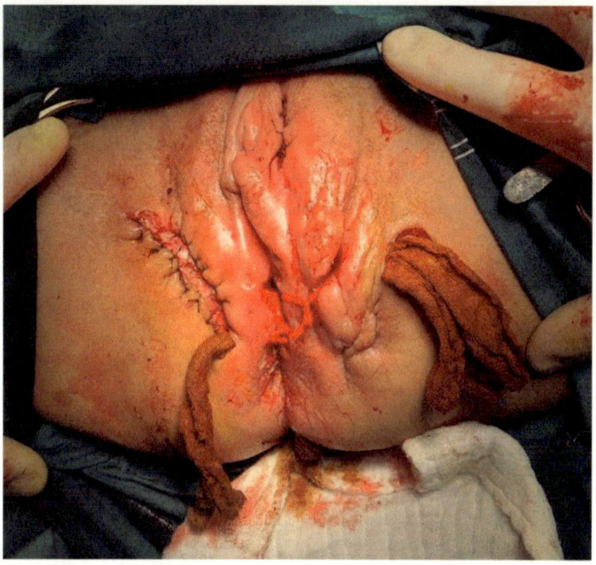

Figure 11.
Perianal form of Crohn's disease in female patient: multiple treatment methods combined (fistulotomy with marsupialization, seton placement, VAAFT).

studied to less invasively induce fistula healing while maintaining fecal continence. When we discuss surgical treatment of complex anal fistulas in Crohn's disease, the goal should be to ameliorate symptoms associated with this kind of fistulas and to improve patients' quality of life. Although, various endoscopic and surgical techniques exist, there is no gold-standard treatment strategy for patients with perianal fistulas [44, 47, 75, 76].

Treatment of Crohn's disease-associated anal fistula should always be multidisciplinary including surgeons, radiologists and gastroenterologists with the use of antibiotics, immunosuppressors and anti-inflammatory agents [77–81].

General principles in the treatment of this condition are underlined here, but the treatment of an anal form of Crohn's disease is a complex topic, requiring a chapter on its own.

7. Discussion and conclusion

The problem of anal continence presents a big obstacle when trying to treat anal fistula. It is of paramount importance to avoid any continence disturbances which in itself presents a hurdle to implementing more successful but invasive procedures regarding the anal sphincter mechanism. The solution might lie in a relatively new paradigm that puts intersphincteric space as a likely culprit to fistula recurrence or nonhealing, and subsequent shift in surgical approach. These new approaches still require multicentric verifications to be implemented as a mainstream treatment option.

Overall, novel approaches in anal fistula treatment, while not entirely successful in all of the patients, offer a significant increase in patients' quality of life, and allow for repeated surgical procedures if the initial operation fails at no expense on the anal sphincter.

While various researchers made different molecular research on anal fistula that increased our understanding of fundamental pathologic mechanisms, still no findings translate into clinical practice in the sense that they made any difference on already existing surgical approaches.

The most widespread classification of fistulas are somewhat inadequate and do not transfer well to clinical situations. Parks classification may describe the relation of the anal fistula to anal sphincter muscles but does not distinguish between simple and complex fistulas. St. James University Hospital classification also doesn't seem relatable to the clinical situations in the era of sphincter preserving techniques. A possible solution to this may be Garg classification that still needs confirmatory commentaries from other colorectal surgeons and proctologists.

Anal fistulas in Crohn's disease present a different challenge. With current surgical solutions, we cannot hope to cure the condition but rather to ameliorate symptoms. Medical therapy in combination with surgical solutions can significantly reduce the severity of the disease and even hope to eradicate it completely.

The anal fistula condition remains a daunting task for the surgeon and a strenuous malady for the patient. Even though recent years brought advancements in the form of sphincter preserving techniques, which greatly improved treatment options, still no golden standard for anal fistula treatment exists. This problem still seems unlikely to resolve given the heterogeneity of pathology unless a radically different approach or breakthrough isn't achieved.

Author details

Damir Karlović*, Dorian Kršul, Ante Jerković, Đordano Bačić and Marko Zelić
Clinical Hospital Center Rijeka, Rijeka, Croatia

*Address all correspondence to: damir.karlovic@yahoo.com

References

[1] Hamalainen KP, Sainio AP. Incidence of fistulas after drainage of acute anorectal abscesses. Diseases of the Colon and Rectum. 1998;**41**:1357-1361

[2] Mappes HJ, Farthmann EH. Anal Abscess and Fistula. Zuckschwardt: Munich; 2001

[3] Parks AG, Gordon PH, Hardcastle JD. A classification of fistula-in-ano. The British Journal of Surgery. 1976;**63**:1-12

[4] Atkin GK, Martins J, Tozer P, Ranchod P, Phillips RKS. For many high anal fistulas, lay open is still a good option. Techniques in Coloproctology. 2011;**15**(2):143-150

[5] Ritchie RD, Sackier JM, Hodde JP. Incontinence rates after cutting seton treatment for anal fistula. Colorectal Disease. 2009;**11**(6):564-571

[6] Lockhart-Mummery JP. Discussion on fistula-in-ano. Proceedings of the Royal Society of Medicine. 1929;**22**:1331-1358

[7] Seow-Choen F, Nicholls RJ. Anal fistula. British Journal of Surgery. 1992;**79**(3):197-205

[8] Garg P. Transanal opening of intersphincteric space (TROPIS)—A new procedure to treat high complex anal fistula. International Journal of Surgery. 2017;**40**:130-134

[9] Garg P. A new understanding of the principles in the management of complex anal fistula. Medical Hypotheses. 2019;**132**:109329

[10] van Onkelen RS, Gosselink MP, van Meurs M, Melief MJ, Schouten WR, Laman JD. Pro-inflammatory cytokines in cryptoglandular anal fistulas. Techniques in Coloproctology. 2016;**20**:619-625

[11] Tozer PJ. Clinical and Experimental Studies in Idiopathic and Crohn's-Related Anal Fistula. 2012. Ph.D. Thesis, Imperial College London

[12] Crespi M, Colombo F, Foschi D. Surgical examination under anesthesia. In: G TMaM. Imaging of Perianal Inflammatory Diseases. Italia: Springer-Verlag; 2013. pp. 67-74

[13] Halligan S, Stoker J. Imaging of fistula in ano. Radiology. 2006;**239**(1):18-33

[14] Ratto C, Grillo E, Parello A, et al. Endoanal ultrasound-guided surgery for anal fistula. Endoscopy. 2005;**37**(8):722-728

[15] Tantiphlachiva K, Sahakitrungruang C, Pattanaarun J, et al. Effects of preoperative endoanal ultrasound on functional outcome after anal fistula surgery. BMJ Open Gastroenterology. 2019;**6**:1-9

[16] West RL, Dwarkasing S, Felt-Bersma RJ, et al. Hydrogen peroxide-enhanced three-dimensional endoanal ultrasonography and endoanal magnetic resonance imaging in evaluating perianal fistulas: Agreement and patient preference. European Journal of Gastroenterology & Hepatology. 2004;**16**:1319-1324

[17] Lunniss PJ, Armstrong P, Barker PG, et al. Magnetic resonance imaging of anal fistulae. Lancet. 1992;**340**:394-396

[18] Maier AG, Funovics MA, Kreuzer SH, et al. Evaluation of perianal sepsis: Comparison of anal endosonography

and magnetic resonance imaging. Journal of Magnetic Resonance Imaging. 2001;**14**(3):254-260

[19] Buchanan GN, Halligan S, Bartram CI, et al. Clinical examination, endosonography, and MR imaging in preoperative assessment of fistula in ano: Comparison with outcome-based reference standard. Radiology. 2004;**233**(3):674-681

[20] Morris J, Spencer JA, Ambrose NS. MR imaging classification of perianal fistulas and its implications for patient management. Radiographics. 2000;**20**(3):623-635

[21] Horsthuis K, Lavini C, Bipat S, et al. Perianal Crohn disease: Evaluation of dynamic contrast-enhanced MR imaging as an indicator of disease activity. Radiology. 2009;**251**(2):380-387

[22] Meinero P, Mori L. Video-assisted anal fistula treatment (VAAFT): A novel sphincter-saving procedure for treating complex anal fistulas. Techniques in Coloproctology. 2011;**15**(4):417-422

[23] Limura E, Giordano P. Modern management of anal fistula. World Journal of Gastroenterology. 2015;**21**(1):12-20

[24] Westerterp M, Volkers NA, Poolman RW, van Tets WF, et al. Practice parameters for the treatment of perianal abscess and fistula-in-ano (revised). Diseases of the Colon and Rectum. 2005;**48**:1337-1342

[25] Mei Z, Wang Q, Zhang Y, et al. Risk Factors for Recurrence after anal fistula surgery: A meta-analysis. International Journal of Surgery. 2019;**69**:153-164

[26] Kršul D, Karlović D, Bačić Đ, Zelić M. Sphincter Preserving Techniques in Anal Fistula Treatment. In: JCBe a, editor. Current Topics in Colorectal Surgery. Rijeka: IntechOpen; 2021

[27] Topalov I, Markov G, Kirov G. Fistula-in-ano treatment a modo Jonesko using brace. Khirurgiia (Sofiia). 2009;**2-3**:38-40

[28] Vogel JD, Johnson EK, Morris AM, Paquette IM, Saclarides TJ, Feingold DL, et al. Clinical practice guideline for the management of anorectal abscess, fistula-in-ano, and rectovaginal fistula. Diseases of the Colon and Rectum. 2016;**59**(12):1117-1133

[29] Göttgens KW, Janssen PT, Heemskerk J, et al. Long-term outcome of low perianal fistulas treated by fistulotomy: A multicenter study. International Journal of Colorectal Disease. 2015;**30**:213-219

[30] Garg P. Assessing validity of existing fistula-in-ano classifications in a cohort of 848 operated and MRI-assessed anal fistula patients—Cohort study. Annals of Medicine and Surgery. 2020;**59**:122-126

[31] Xu Y, Liang S, Tang W. Meta-analysis of randomized clinical trials comparing fistulectomy versus fistulotomy for low anal fistula. Springerplus. 2016;**5**(1):1722

[32] Mitalas LE, van Wijk JJ, Gosselink MP, Doornebosch P, Zimmerman DD, Schouten WR. Seton drainage prior to transanal advancement flap repair: Useful or not? International Journal of Colorectal Disease. 2010;**25**: 1499-1502

[33] Hong KD, Kang S, Kalaskar S, Wexner SD. Ligation of intersphincteric fistula tract (LIFT) to treat anal fistula: Systematic review and meta-analysis. Techniques in Coloproctology. 2014;**18**(8):685-691

[34] Voon KKT, Shanwani A, Mazlan KM, Zakaria Z. Modified-2-staged

fistulectomy with sphincter repair (m2fisr) procedure for transphincteric fistula-in-ano: A modified surgical approach. Brunei International Medical Journal. 2020;**16**:117-123

[35] Giamundo P, Esercizio L, Geraci M, Tibaldi L, et al. Fistula tract Laser Closure (FiLaC): Long-term results and new operative strategies. Techniques in Coloproctology. 2015;**19**:449-453

[36] Ommer A, Herold A, Joos AK, Schmidt C, et al. Gore BioA Fistula Plug in the treatment of high anal fistulas—initial results from a German multicenter-study. GMS German Medical Science. 2012;**10**:1-17

[37] McGee MF, Champagne BJ, Stulberg JJ, Reynolds H, et al. Tract length predicts successful closure with anal fistula plug in cryptoglandular fistulas. Diseases of the Colon & Rectum. 2010;**53**:1116-1120

[38] Zelić M, Karlović D, Kršul D, Bačić Đ, Warusavitarne J. Video-assisted anal fistula treatment (VAAFT) for treatment of complex cryptoglandular anal fistulas with 2 years follow up period—Our experience. Journal of Laparoendoscopic & Advanced Surgical Techniques. Part A. 2020;**30**(12):13

[39] Rojanasakul A. LIFT procedure: A simplified technique for fistula-in-ano. Techniques in Coloproctology. 2009;**13**(3):237-240

[40] Pérez-Lara FJ, Moreno Serrano A, Ulecia Moreno J, et al. Platelet-rich fibrin sealant as a treatment for complex perianal fistulas: A multicentre study. Journal of Gastrointestinal Surgery. 2015;**19**:360-368

[41] Balciscueta Z, Uribe N, Balciscueta I, et al. Rectal advancement flap for the treatment of complex cryptoglandular anal fistulas: A systematic review and meta-analysis. International Journal of Colorectal Disease. 2017;**32**:599-609

[42] Ozuner G, Hull TL, Cartmill J, Fazio VW. Long-term analysis of the use of transanal rectal advancement flaps for complicated anorectal/vaginal fistulas. Diseases of the Colon and Rectum. 1996;**39**:10-14

[43] Emile SH, Khan SM, Adejumo A, Koroye O. Ligation of intersphincteric fistula tract (LIFT) in treatment of anal fistula: An updated systematic review, meta-analysis, and meta-regression of the predictors of failure. Surgery. 2020;**167**(2):484-492

[44] Schwandner O. Video-assisted anal fistula treatment (VAAFT) combined with advancement flap repair in Crohn's disease. Techniques in Coloproctology. 2013;**17**(2):221-225

[45] Walega P, Romaniszyn M, Nowak W. VAAFT: A new minimally invasive method in the diagnostics and treatment of anal fistulas—Initial results. Polski Przeglad Chirurgiczny. 2014;**86**(1):7-10

[46] Emile SH, Elfeki H, Shalaby M, Sakr A. A Systematic review and meta-analysis of the efficacy and safety of video-assisted anal fistula treatment (VAAFT). Surgical Endoscopy. 2018;**32**(4):2084-2093

[47] Adegbola SO, Sahnan K, Tozer PJ, Strouhal R, Hart AL, Lung PFC, et al. Symptom amelioration in Crohn's perianal fistulas using video-assisted anal fistula treatment (VAAFT). Journal of Crohn's & Colitis. 2018;**12**(9):1067-1072

[48] García-Aguilar J, Davey CS, Le CT, Lowry AC, Rothenberger DA. Patient satisfaction after surgical treatment for fistula-in-ano. Diseases of the Colon and Rectum. 2000;**43**(9):1206-1212

[49] Dubsky PC, Stift A, Friedl J, Teleky B, Herbst F. Endorectal advancement flaps in the treatment of high anal fistula of cryptoglandular origin: Fullthickness vs. mucosal-rectum flaps. Diseases of the Colon and Rectum. 2008;**51**:852-857

[50] Khafagy W, Omar W, El Nakeeb A, Fouda E, Yousef M, Farid M. Treatment of anal fistulas by partial rectal wall advancement flap or mucosal advancement flap: A prospective randomized study. International Journal of Surgery. 2010;**8**:321-325

[51] Schouten WR, Zimmerman DD, Briel JW. Transanal advancement flap repair of transsphincteric fistulas. Diseases of the Colon and Rectum. 1999;**42**:1419-1422

[52] Zimmerman DD, Delemarre JB, Gosselink MP, et al. Smoking affects the outcome of transanal mucosal advancement flap repair of transsphincteric fistulas. The British Journal of Surgery. 2003;**90**:351-354

[53] Ellis CN, Clark S. Effect of tobacco smoking on advancement flap repair of complex anal fistulas. Diseases of the Colon and Rectum. 2007;**50**:459-463

[54] Schwandner O. Obesity is a negative predictor of success after surgery for complex anal fistula. BMC Gastroenterology. 2011;**11**(61):1-5

[55] Karlović D, Kršul D, Bačić Đ, Zelić M. Video-assisted anal fistula treatment in combination with ligation of the intersphincteric fistula tract in the treatment of complex transsphincteric fistulas—A video vignette. Colorectal Disease. 2020;**22**(9):1204-1201

[56] La Torre M, Lisi G, D'Agostino E, et al. Lift and VAAFT for high trans-sphincteric anal fistula: A single center retrospective analysis. International Journal of Colorectal Disease. 2020;**35**(6):1149-1153

[57] Yao Y-B, Xiao C-F, Wang Q-T. VAAFT plus FiLaC™: A combined procedure for complex anal fistula. Techniques in Coloproctology. 2021;**25**:977-979

[58] Ellis CN. Outcomes with the use of bioprosthetic grafts to reinforce the ligation of the intersphincteric fistula tract (BioLIFT procedure) for the management of complex anal fistulas. Diseases of the Colon and Rectum. 2010;**53**(10):1361

[59] Han JG, Yi BQ, Wang ZJ, Zheng Y, Cui JJ, Yu XQ, et al. Ligation of the intersphincteric fistula tract plus a bioprosthetic anal fistula plug (LIFTPlug): A new technique for fistula-in ano. Colorectal Disease. 2013;**15**(5):582

[60] Sileri P, Boehm G, Franceschilli L, et al. Collagen matrix injection combined with flap repair for complex anal fistula. Colorectal Disease. 2012;**14**:24

[61] Ratto C, Litta F, Donisi L, Parello A. Fistulotomy or fistulectomy and primary sphincteroplasty for anal fistula (FIPS): A systematic review. Techniques in Coloproctology. 2015;**19**(7):391-400

[62] Ommer A, Herold A, Berg E, et al. German S3 guidelines: Anal abscess and fistula (second revised version). Langenbeck's Archives of Surgery. 2017;**402**(2):191-201

[63] Bai MY, Wang CW, Wang JY, Lin MF, Chan WP. Threedimensional structure and cytokine distribution of platelet-rich fibrin. Clinics (São Paulo, Brazil). 2017;**72**:116-124

[64] Eppley BL, Woodell GE, Higgins J. Platelet quantification and growth factor

analysis from platelet-rich plasma: Implications for wound healing. Plastic and Reconstructive Surgery. 2004;**114**:1502-1508

[65] Van der Hagen SJ, Baeten CG, Soeters PB, van Gemert WG. Autologous platelet-derived growth factors (platelet-rich plasma) as an adjunct to mucosal advancement flap in high cryptoglandular perianal fistulae: A pilot study. Colorectal Disease. 2011;**13**:215-218

[66] Göttgens KW, Vening W, van der Hagen SJ, et al. Longterm results of mucosal advancement flap combined with platelet rich plasma for high cryptoglandular perianal fistulas. Diseases of the Colon & Rectum. 2014;**57**(22):223-227

[67] Göttgens KWA, Smeets RR, Stassen LPS, et al. Treatment of Crohn's disease-related high perianal fistulas combining the mucosa advancement flap with platelet-rich plasma: A pilot study. Techniques in Coloproctology. 2015;**19**:455-459

[68] Moreno-Serrano A, García-Díaz JJ, Ferrer-Márquez M, et al. Using autologous platelet-rich plasma for the treatment of complex fistulas. Revista Española de Enfermedades Digestivas. 2016;**108**:123-128

[69] Safar B, Sands D. Perianal Crohn's disease. Clinics in Colon and Rectal Surgery. 2007;**20**(4):282-293

[70] Kotze PG, Shen B, Lightner A, et al. Modern management of perianal fistulas in Crohn's disease: Future directions. Gut. 2018;**67**(8):1181-1194

[71] Sica GS, Di Carlo S, Tema G, et al. Treatment of perianal fistula in Crohn's disease. World Journal of Gastroenterology. 2014;**20**(37): 13205-13210

[72] Marzo M, Felice C, Pugliese D, et al. Management of perianal fistulas in Crohn's disease: An up-to-date review. World Journal of Gastroenterology. 2015;**21**(5):1394-1403

[73] Sandborn WJ, Fazio VW, Feagan BG, Hanauer SB. American gastroenterological association clinical practice committee. AGA technical review on perianal Crohn's disease. Gastroenterology. 2003;**125**(5):1508-1530

[74] Bubbers EJ, Cologne KG. Management of complex anal fistulas. Clinics in Colon and Rectal Surgery. 2016;**29**(1):43-49

[75] Moy J, Bodzin J. Carbon dioxide laser ablation of perianal fistulas in patients with Crohn's disease: Experience with 27 patients. American Journal of Surgery. 2006;**191**(3):424-427

[76] Wilhelm A. A new technique for sphincter-preserving anal fistula repair using a novel radial emitting laser probe. Techniques in Coloproctology. 2011;**15**(4):445-449

[77] Asteria CR, Ficari F, Bagnoli S, et al. Treatment of perianal fistulas in Crohn's disease by local injection of antibody to TNF-alpha accounts for a favourable clinical response in selected cases: A pilot study. Scandinavian Journal of Gastroenterology. 2006;**41**(9):1064-1072

[78] Alessandroni L, Kohn A, Cosintino R, et al. Local injection of infliximab in severe fistulating perianal Crohn's disease: An open uncontrolled study. Techniques in Coloproctology. 2011;**15**(4):407-412

[79] Tonelli F, Giudici F, Asteria CR. Effectiveness and safety of local adalimumab injection in patients with fistulizing perianal Crohn's disease: A pilot study. Diseases of the Colon and Rectum. 2012;**55**(8):870-875

[80] Khorrami S, Ginard D, Marín-Jiménez I, et al. Ustekinumab for the treatment of refractory Crohn's disease: The Spanish experience in a large multicentre open-label cohort. Inflammatory Bowel Diseases. 2016;**22**(6):1662-1669

[81] Sandborn WJ, Feagan BG, Rutgeerts P, et al. GEMINI 2 Study Group. Vedolizumab as induction and maintenance therapy for Crohn's disease. The New England Journal of Medicine. 2013;**369**(8):711-721

Chapter 2

Sphincterotomy is the Gold-Standard Treatment of Chronic Anal Fissure: But How Should it be Done?

Bengi Balci, Sezai Leventoglu and Bulent Mentes

Abstract

A chronic anal fissure is one of the most encountered anorectal diseases in the clinical practice of general surgery. After all the medical therapies have failed, lateral internal sphincterotomy is still the main-stay treatment for chronic anal fissure. The optimal and standardized sphincterotomy has the utmost importance in preventing postoperative incontinence and recurrence, which are consequences of either extreme or insufficient sphincterotomy. Therefore, the lateral internal sphincterotomy technique has been evolved within years with the initial proposition of controlled-sphincterotomy and improvement of this technique with the addition of sphincterotomy up to the dentate line. This chapter focuses on the chronic anal fissure in the era of spasm-controlled lateral internal sphincterotomy.

Keywords: acute anal fissure, chronic anal fissure, internal sphincterotomy, spasm-controlled, incontinence

1. Introduction

An anal fissure is one of the most encountered anorectal diseases by general surgeons, although the true prevalence is unknown [1]. It is described as a tear developing in the squamous epithelium of the anoderm and is located between the dentate line and the anal verge [2].

This condition is often related to chronic constipation and difficulty of defecation and rarely can result from Crohn's disease, tuberculosis, and Acquired Immune Deficiency Syndrome (AIDS). The most common location of the fissure is the posterior midline (90%), followed by the anterior midline (1–10%), and lateral (1%). Lateral fissures can be associated with an underlying disease and should be thoroughly investigated. Typical symptoms are anal pain during defecation, bleeding, pruritus, and soiling.

An anal fissure can be described as acute and chronic according to the duration of symptoms. An acute fissure is a superficial lesion that usually occurs after constipation/diarrhea and can be healed with conservative management in 4 to 6 weeks. In contrast, chronic anal fissure is a deeper lesion surrounded by scar tissue caused by chronic inflammation. Chronic inflammation can cause skin tags in the anoderm adjacent to the fissure and hypertrophic papilla in the anal canal. Medical treatment is often ineffective for chronic fissures, and the patient's symptoms are prolonged to 6 to 8 weeks.

2. Pathogenesis

The triggering factor is usually thought to be trauma to the anoderm from the passage of hard stool or chronic irritation from diarrhea, but the exact etiology of anal fissure remains unclear. Two major hypotheses have been proposed regarding the development of chronic fissures: the presence of hypertonicity in the internal anal sphincter and relatively decreased tissue perfusion in the posterior midline [3–5] (**Figure 1**).

It has also been suggested that hypertonicity may result in pressure on the perpendicular vessels in the internal anal sphincter muscle and may compromise perfusion to the posterior midline even more [6]. Therefore, most of the medical and surgical treatments have been developed to decrease the internal sphincter's tonicity. Regardless of these hypotheses, hypertonicity may not be found in all patients with chronic anal fissures. Also, constipation and hard bowel movements have only been reported in 13% of these patients [7, 8].

3. Clinical presentation and diagnosis

Patients usually present with moderate to severe anal pain, described as "like passing broken glass," aggravated by defecation, and lasts several minutes to hours afterward [9]. Although bleeding occurs less commonly in anal fissures than hemorrhoidal diseases, patients may notice a small amount of bright-red blood on the toilet paper resulting from chronic ulceration in the epithelium (**Figure 2**).

Based on these predominant symptoms, an acute or chronic anal fissure can be diagnosed during the first interrogation. Nevertheless, the clinician should always consider an underlying cause of chronic constipation related to the fissure, such as rectocele, diverticular disease, and colorectal cancer.

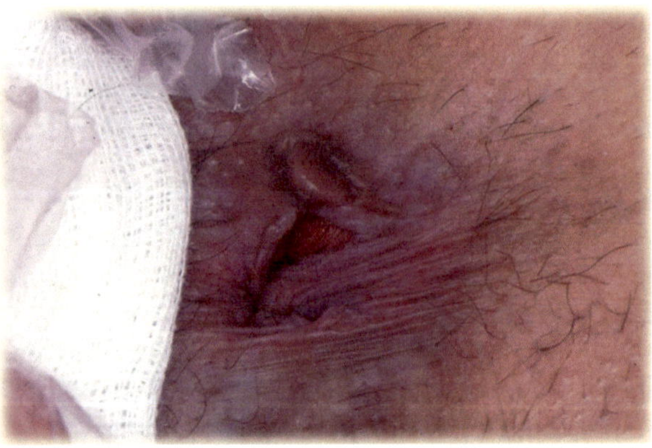

Figure 1.
Operative image of a patient with chronic anal fissure shows the spasm in the sphincter complex even under sedation.

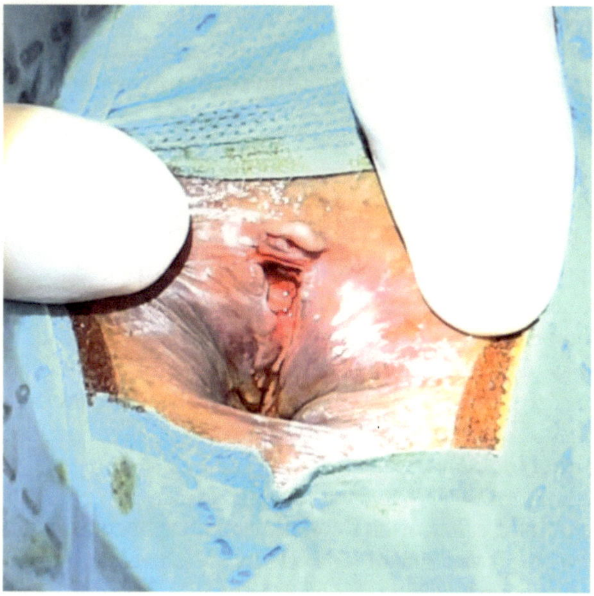

Figure 2.
Chronic anal fissure presenting with bleeding.

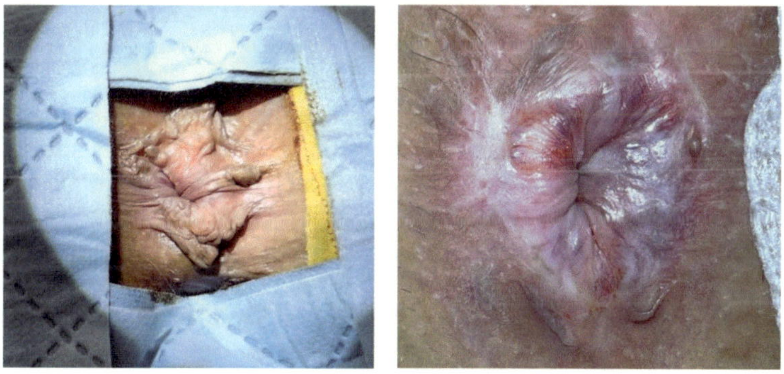

Figure 3.
Physical examination involves the inspection of number of fissures and the presence of skin tags. a) Multiple skin tags b) multiple chronic fissures in the posterior, lateral, and anterior of the anal canal.

On physical examination, the location, depth, and the number of fissures should be noted in addition to the presence of skin tags and chronic inflammation surrounding the lesion (**Figure 3**). Initially, a digital rectal examination may not be performed due to severe pain in an acute anal fissure; in that case, a detailed examination under anesthesia with anoscope and rectosigmoidoscopy may be required [10].

4. Non-operative management

Usual recommendations for acute anal fissure include increased fiber and fluid ingestion, the use of local anesthetic ointments, warm daily sitz-bath, and stool softeners. Although almost half of the acute fissures heal with these conservative treatments, the success rate is as low as 30% in chronic fissures [10–12]. Given the cost-effectiveness and potential risk of incontinence with surgery, international guidelines still recommend topical and botulinum toxin injection as first-line therapy.

4.1 Nitrates

The mechanism of nitrates is based on the release of nitric oxide, which influences the relaxation of the internal anal sphincter muscle [13, 14]. Its commonly used form is glyceryl trinitrate (GTN) in 0.2–0.4% doses, and it is applied topically two to three times a day. The topical application of GTN has been reported to decrease anal resting pressures and promote healing in anal fissure compared to placebo; however, 50% of patients' disease has recurred in the long term [11]. Major side-effects and reasons for discontinuing the treatment are headaches and light-headedness [15, 16].

4.2 Calcium-channel blockers

Topical application of calcium-channel blockers has been proven to effectively heal anal fissures with a lower risk of side effects [17]. Topically applied 0.5% nifedipine has been found to have healing rates of 93% in a duration of 19-month follow-up [18]. Also, Khan et al. have proved significantly higher healing rates (80.4%) with 2% topical diltiazem compared to GTN application [19]. Similarly, 0.5% topical minoxidil has been shown as equally effective as diltiazem [20].

4.3 Botulinum toxin

Botulinum toxin is an exotoxin produced by *Clostridium botulinum,* and its injection prevents the release of acetylcholine from the presynaptic nerve terminals, thus results resulting in temporary muscle paralysis. The first use of botulinum toxin in treating anal fissure was described in 1993 by Jost and Schimrigk [21, 22].

Although there is no standardized treatment with botulinum toxin regarding the dose and injection site, it is commonly injected directly into the internal anal sphincter on either side of the midline, with doses varying from 5 to 100 units [23, 24]. Pilkington et al. have revealed no significant differences between unilateral and bilateral injections in healing and fissure pain relief in a randomized prospective study [25]. In a retrospective review of patients who have been treated with high-dose (80–100 IU) and low-dose (20–40 IU) botulinum toxin, recurrence rates have been found significantly lower in a high-dose group during a mean follow-up of 25 months [26]. However, a meta-analysis has demonstrated no dose-dependent efficiency [27].

Several comparative studies have investigated the healing rates and symptomatic relief after botulinum toxin and topical agents [28–32]. Sajid et al. have shown that botulinum toxin injection has had similar healing rates with GTN but fewer side effects [33]. Also, another study has demonstrated that overall cure rates have been similar between diltiazem (53%), GTN (54%), and botulinum toxin (51%) [34]. A guideline published in 2017 has stated that botulinum toxin injection has similar results with topical agents as first-line therapy and modest improvement in healing rates as second-line therapy following treatment with topical agents [10].

The significant drawbacks of botulinum toxin injection are the risk of incontinence and its temporary effectiveness that usually lasts 3–6 months [35, 36]. Moreover, there are still unanswered questions: the following step when botulinum toxin fails if the second injection should be performed, the interval for repeat injection, and the timing of surgery. A recent study has discussed some of those issues among colorectal surgeons on practice parameters of botulinum toxin treatment [37]. It has been shown that more than half of the clinicians perform the second injection in case of persistence of symptoms and recurrence, and the interval for repeat injection has usually been more than 2 months.

5. Surgical treatment of chronic anal fissure

Traditionally, lateral internal sphincterotomy (LIS) has been the gold-standard treatment for chronic anal fissure [38]. This technique decreases the pressure caused by the internal anal sphincter hypertonicity, normalizes the perfusion on the anoderm, alleviates the pain, and promotes fissure healing [3] (**Figure 4**). With trends toward topical agents and botulinum toxin injection, several studies have been conducted to compare the outcomes of these treatment methods [39–42]. A randomized controlled trial by Mentes et al. has revealed that LIS is superior to botulinum toxin injection regarding healing and recurrence in the long term [43]. Similar results have been obtained by Arroyo et al., 1-year healing rates with botulinum toxin and LIS were 45% and 93%, respectively [44].

5.1 Techniques of lateral internal sphincterotomy

The main issue with LIS has been the risk of incontinence [45]. Garg et al. have reported incontinence rates as 14% during a follow-up of 2 years [46]. In this study, most patients complained of flatus incontinence (9%), followed by soiling/seepage (6%), incontinence to liquid stool (0.91%), and solid stool (0.63%).

Determining risk factors for incontinence after LIS include the history of vaginal delivery, female patients, anteriorly located fissures, age over 40–50, concomitant anorectal procedures (hemorrhoidectomy), and presence of incontinence in pre operative setting [46]. The effects of LIS on quality of life have been evaluated by using the Gastrointestinal Quality of Life Index (GQLI) and the Fecal Incontinence Quality of Life Scale (FIQLS) in a 1-year follow-up [47]. Moreover, GQLI scores have significantly improved after LIS, and only three patients (1.2%) experienced deterioration in FIQLS scores.

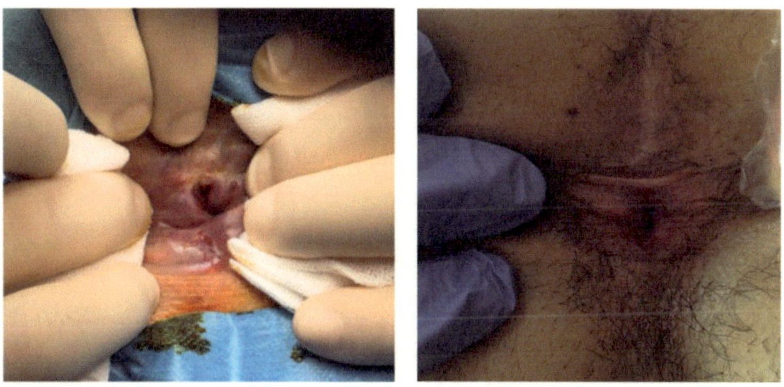

Figure 4.
Healing of the chronic anal fissure. a) Preoperative image, b) postoperative 6-month image.

Although LIS has been performing for over decades, there has not been a standardized technique, and with increased reporting of incontinence, the search for optimal sphincterotomy regarding the level and degree of sphincter division has commenced. In the following sections, variations in sphincterotomy techniques will be discussed.

5.1.1 Open lateral internal sphincterotomy

The open technique involves a radial incision made on the intersphincteric groove and the dissection and division of the internal sphincter muscle to the level of the dentate line. The incision is usually left open for drainage (**Figure 5**).

In a prospective randomized study, delayed healing and higher postoperative pain scores have been found in the open technique group [48]. Similar results have been obtained by Pernkoft and Kortbeek et al., who have reported lower complication rates with the closed technique [49, 50].

5.1.2 Closed lateral internal sphincterotomy

The closed technique involves the digital palpation of the sphincter complex, simultaneously inserting a blade into the intersphincteric groove and dividing the

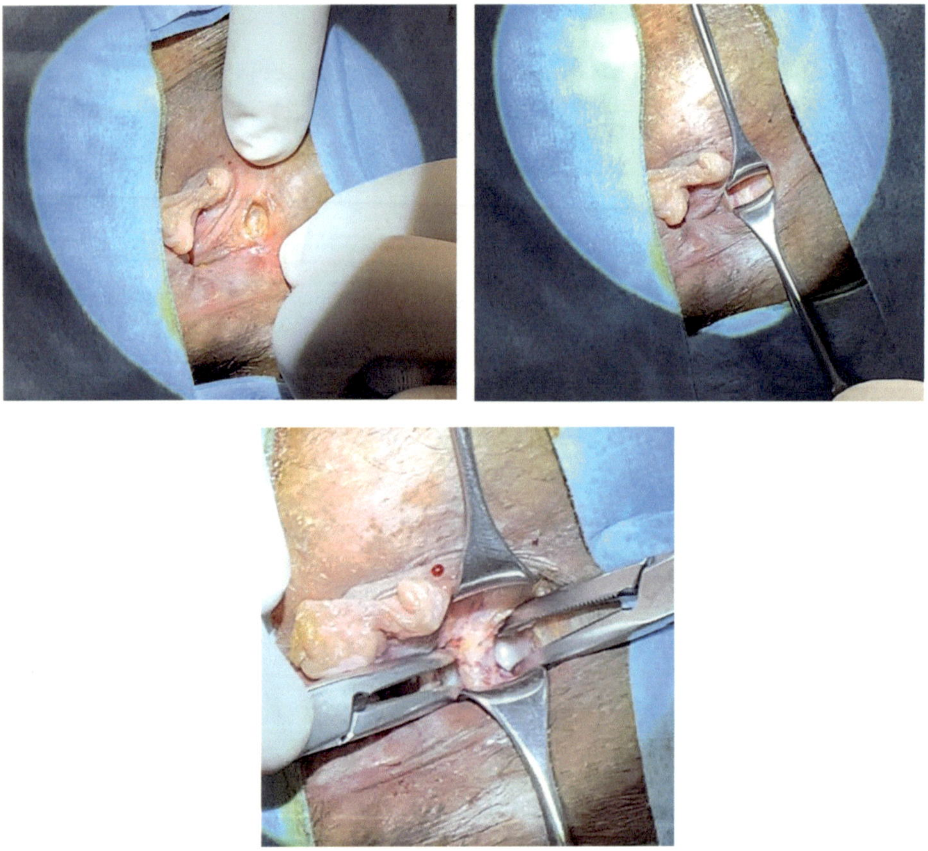

Figure 5.
The steps of open lateral internal sphincterotomy. a) the circumferential incision is made in the intersphincteric groove, b) deepening the dissection with the help of retractors, c) the division of the internal sphincter muscle.

internal sphincter by moving the blade medially. The expected rate of division is 1/3 to 1/2 of the internal sphincter muscle.

Many authors have reported that the closed technique is effective and safe with a similar cure and fewer complication rates [51, 52]. In contrast, Wiley et al. has demonstrated similar incontinence rates between open and closed techniques, although overall, 6.8% of incontinence rates have been detected during a follow-up of 52 weeks [53]. Based on these contradicted results, it has been suggested that rather than an open or closed approach, the extent of sphincterotomy may influence the rates of incontinence and healing [54].

5.1.3 Radial vs. circumferential incision in lateral internal sphincterotomy

According to the surgeons' experience and preference, open sphincterotomy can be performed with radial or circumferential incisions. Ersoz et al. has reported that the circumferential incision is associated with shorter healing time and fewer itching sensations than radial incisions [55]. Similar results about reduced time for wound healing with circumferential incision have also been proven by Kang et al. [56]. Both authors have suggested that the fecal material creates an outward force vector resulting in dilatation of the anal canal associated with more dehiscence in the radial incision.

5.1.4 Extent of sphincterotomy

Another attempt to decrease incontinence rates has been the proposal of performing sphincterotomy up to the height of the fissure apex instead of to the dentate line [57]. This technique initially showed high healing rates with significantly lower incontinence rates [58]. However, long-term follow-up results have demonstrated higher rates of treatment failure and slower effects on healing [59]. In another study evaluating the recurrence/persistence of fissure and incontinence rates, endoanal ultrasonography was performed after percutaneous and open sphincterotomy [60]. It has been confirmed that open and complete sphincterotomy is associated with lower recurrence rates but increased incontinence, while partial and percutaneous sphincterotomy has resulted in persistence and recurrence of the fissure. These results have supported that sphincterotomy should be complete but shorter, whether percutaneous or open sphincterotomy is performed.

Furthermore, the extent of sphincterotomy and its association with incontinence have been investigated between female patients and the control group by performing three-dimensional anal ultrasonography [61]. The extent of sphincterotomy has been directly related to incontinence, and it should be less than 25% of the total sphincter length (less than 1 cm in females) (**Figure 6**). Interestingly, this study has also demonstrated a significant decrease in anal resting pressure, whereas the maximum squeeze pressure has remained similar to preoperative measurements. A recent study has also reported supporting findings for dividing the internal sphincter by about 20% in female patients [62].

5.1.5 Ultramodified internal sphincterotomy

Sungurtekin et al. has described a new technique called ultra-modified internal sphincterotomy, which involves an incision made in the base of the posterior fissure, identification of the internal and external sphincter under direct vision, division of previously measured 1 cm of internal sphincter bundle [63].

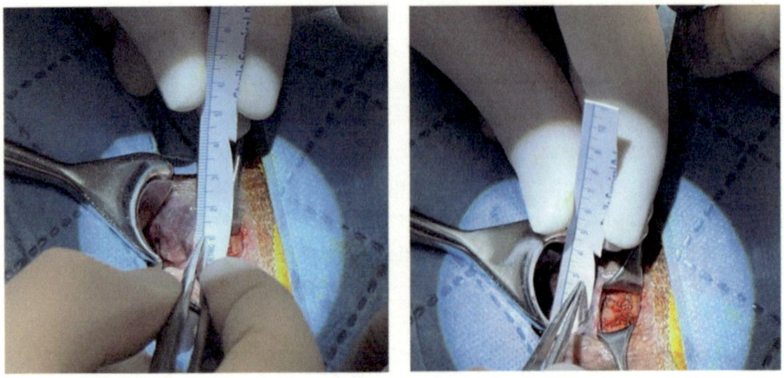

Figure 6.
Measurement of sphincterotomy. a) Sphincterotomy is measured as 1 cm from the anal verge, b) the distance of sphincterotomy to the dentate line is shown as 2 cm.

They have reported the results of this technique in comparison to the closed sphincterotomy. The anal resting pressures have decreased in both study groups; however, the decline in pressures has lasted for 24 months in closed technique and is attributed to iatrogenic damage in the internal anal sphincter. Moreover, the patient satisfaction and recovery rates have been higher in the ultramodified sphincterotomy group.

5.1.6 Spasm-controlled sphincterotomy

Previous findings have created a whole new perspective in the technique of sphincterotomy, suggesting that the sphincter division should be made in a tailored fashion by considering the differences in genders, anal calibers, and anal resting pressures.

A tailored, spasm-controlled sphincterotomy term by performing sphincterotomy according to the anal caliber was first proposed by Cho et al. [64]. A prospective comparative study has investigated the outcomes of spasm-controlled and up to the fissure

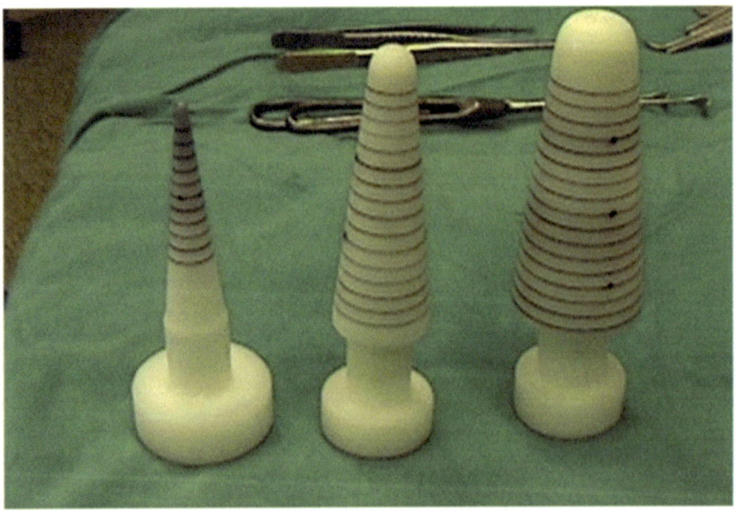

Figure 7.
Anal calibrators are used to measure the anal caliber in the spasm-controlled technique. Small, medium and large calibrators are in the size of 5–15, 15–30, and 27–43 mm, respectively [65].

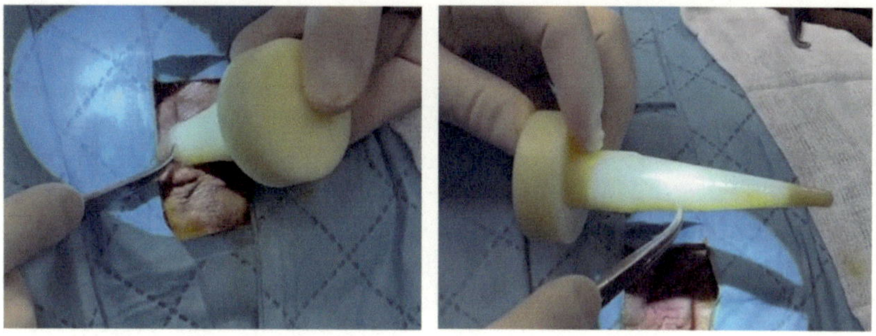

Figure 8.
In the spasm-controlled technique, anal calibrations are measured before and after sphincterotomy. a) Small anal calibrator is measured as 5–15 mm, b) anal caliber is measured about 12 mm in this patient with chronic anal fissure.

apex sphincterotomy [65]. The spasm-controlled technique was performed by small serial sphincterotomies using an anal calibrator to achieve a 25–30 mm anal caliber, while fissure apex sphincterotomy was performed in a traditional way (**Figure 7**). Not surprisingly, the incontinence rates have been found significantly lower with described technique, and there was no significant difference in treatment failure (**Figure 8**).

6. Tips and tricks

- Local or regional anesthesia are preferred in combination with sedative drugs. Regional anesthesia may be required for patients with high body mass index considering the difficulties in respiration with the prone position.
- Injecting local anesthetics consisting of lidocaine hydrochloride with adrenaline to the incision area enables a blood-free surgical area.
- The prone jack-knife position provides good exposure to the anal canal and sphincter complex.
- Anal caliber is measured with anal calibrators at the initial of the procedure.
- A circumferential 1 cm incision made on the right lateral of the anal canal is the chosen approach. Subcutaneous dissection is performed in the intersphincteric groove with the help of small retractors.
- The lateral internal sphincter muscle is divided under the direct vision as small bites at each time, and the anal caliber is repeatedly measured to obtain a predetermined anal caliber of 25–30 mm.
- The incision is partially closed using continuous 4–0 absorbable sutures.
- Fissurectomy might be performed in addition to sphincterotomy in patients with severe pain and soiling symptoms due to deep scar tissue.
- Large skin tags can also be excised for cosmetic and hygiene issues, if so, one should be avoided to excise a large amount of anoderm.

7. Conclusions

Lateral internal sphincterotomy is still the gold-standard treatment for chronic anal fissures when the first-line and second-line therapies such as topical nitrates, calcium-channel blockers, and botulinum toxin have failed. It is associated with increased healing rates and improved quality of life in patients with anal fissures. Therefore, surgical intervention can even be offered in select patients without first confirming the failure of pharmacological therapies.

The technique of lateral internal sphincterotomy has been evolved over the years in terms of approaches (open/closed), the level of division of the internal sphincter (complete/partial), and the extent of sphincterotomy (to the dentate line/up to the fissure apex). A tailored-fashion sphincterotomy that is based on the individual characteristics of each patient has come upfront in recent years. As a tailored-fashion technique, the spasm-controlled sphincterotomy has been performed as a safe and effective method with low rates of incontinence and treatment failure.

Determining an individualized technique, which involves objective methods to measure the sufficient level of sphincterotomy either by calibrators and a surgical measure or anal ultrasonography and manometry, has the utmost importance in preventing postoperative incontinence, increasing healing rates, and improving quality of life.

Conflict of interest

All authors declare that they have no conflict of interest.

Author details

Bengi Balci[1], Sezai Leventoglu[2*] and Bulent Mentes[3]

1 Department of General Surgery, Ankara Oncology Training and Research Hospital, Ankara, Turkey

2 Department of General Surgery, School of Medicine, Gazi University, Ankara, Turkey

3 Department of General Surgery/Proctology, Memorial Ankara Hospital, Ankara, Turkey

*Address all correspondence to: sezaileventoglu@hotmail.com

References

[1] Fleshman JW. Fissure-in-ano and anal stenosis. In: Becker DE, Wexner SD, editors. Fundamentals of Anorectal Surgery. London: W.B. Saunders; 1998. p. 557

[2] Zaghiyan KN, Fleshner P. Anal fissure. Clinics in Colon and Rectal Surgery. 2011;**24**(1):22-30. DOI: 10.1055/s-0031-1272820

[3] Schouten WR, Briel JW, Aurwerda JJ, De Graaf EJ. Ischaemic nature of anal fissure. The British Journal of Surgery. 1996;**83**:63-65

[4] Utzig MJ, Kroesen AJ, Buhr HJ. Concepts in pathogenesis and treatment of chronic anal fissure: A review of the literature. Journal of Gastroenterology. 2003;**98**:968-974

[5] Lund JN, Scholefield JH. Aetiology and treatment of anal fissure. The British Journal of Surgery. 1996;**83**:1335-1344

[6] Klosterhalfen B, Vogel P, Rixen H, et al. Topography of the inferior rectal artery: A possible cause of chronic, primary anal fissure. Diseases of the Colon and Rectum. 1989;**32**:43-52

[7] Herzig DO, Lu KC. Anal fissure. The Surgical Clinics of North America. 2010;**90**:33-44

[8] Beaty JS, Shashidharan M. Anal fissure. Clinics in Colon and Rectal Surgery. 2016;**29**(1):30-37. DOI: 10.1055/s-0035-1570390

[9] Salati SA. Anal fissure - an extensive update. Polski Przeglad Chirurgiczny. 2021;**93**(4):46-56. DOI: 10.5604/01.3001.0014.7879

[10] Stewart DB Sr, Gaertner W, Glasgow S, Migaly J, Feingold D, Steele SR. Clinical practice guideline for the Management of Anal Fissures. Diseases of the Colon and Rectum. 2017;**60**(1):7-14. DOI: 10.1097/DCR.0000000000000735

[11] Nelson RL, Thomas K, Morgan J, Jones A. Non surgical therapy for anal fissure. Cochrane Database of Systematic Reviews. 2012;**2012**(2):CD003431. DOI: 10.1002/14651858.CD003431.pub3

[12] Boland PA, Kelly ME, Donlon NE, Bolger JC, Larkin JO, Mehigan BJ, et al. Management options for chronic anal fissure: A systematic review of randomised controlled trials. International Journal of Colorectal Disease. 2020;**35**(10):1807-1815. DOI: 10.1007/s00384-020-03699-4

[13] O'Kelly TJ. Nerves that say NO: A new perspective on the human rectoanal inhibitory reflex. Annals of the Royal College of Surgeons of England. 1996;**78**:31-38

[14] Fung HL. Clinical pharmacology of organic nitrates. The American Journal of Cardiology. 1993;**72**(8):9C-13C; discussion 14C-15C. DOI: 10.1016/0002-9149(93)90249-c

[15] Hyman NH, Cataldo PA. Nitroglycerin ointment for anal fissures: Effective treatment or just a headache? Diseases of the Colon and Rectum. 1999;**42**(3):383-385. DOI: 10.1007/BF02236358

[16] Dorfman G, Levitt M, Platell C. Treatment of chronic anal fissure with topical glyceryl trinitrate. Diseases of the Colon and Rectum. 1999;**42**(8):1007-1010. DOI: 10.1007/BF02236692

[17] Jonas M, Speake W, Scholefield JH. Diltiazem heals glyceryl trinitrate-resistant chronic anal fissures: A

prospective study. Diseases of the Colon and Rectum. 2002;**45**(8):1091-1095. DOI: 10.1007/s10350-004-6365-z

[18] Katsinelos P, Papaziogas B, Koutelidakis I, Paroutoglou G, Dimiropoulos S, Souparis A, et al. Topical 0.5% nifedipine vs. lateral internal sphincterotomy for the treatment of chronic anal fissure: Long-term follow-up. International Journal of Colorectal Disease. 2006;**21**(2):179-183. DOI: 10.1007/s00384-005-0766-x

[19] Khan MS, Akbar I, Zeb J, Ahmad S, Khan A. Outcome of 0.2% Glyceryltrinitrate cream versus 2% diltiazem cream in the treatment of chronic anal fissure. Journal of Ayub Medical College, Abbottabad. 2017;**29**(2):280-284

[20] Alvandipour M, Ala S, Khalvati M, Yazdanicharati J, Koulaeinejad N. Topical Minoxidil versus topical diltiazem for chemical Sphincterotomy of chronic anal fissure: A prospective, randomized, double-blind, clinical trial. World Journal of Surgery. 2018;**42**(7):2252-2258. DOI: 10.1007/s00268-017-4449-x

[21] Jost WH, Schimrigk K. Use of botulinum toxin in anal fissure. Diseases of the Colon and Rectum. 1993;**36**(10):974. DOI: 10.1007/BF02050639

[22] Jost WH. Ten years' experience with botulin toxin in anal fissure. International Journal of Colorectal Disease. 2002;**17**(5):298-302. DOI: 10.1007/s00384-002-0398-3

[23] Maria G, Brisinda G, Bentivoglio AR, Cassetta E, Gui D, Albanese A. Botulinum toxin injections in the internal anal sphincter for the treatment of chronic anal fissure: Long-term results after two different dosage regimens. Annals of Surgery. 1998;**228**(5):664-669. DOI: 10.1097/00000658-199811000-00005

[24] Mínguez M, Melo F, Espí A, García-Granero E, Mora F, Lledó S, et al. Therapeutic effects of different doses of botulinum toxin in chronic anal fissure. Diseases of the Colon and Rectum. 1999;**42**(8):1016-1021. DOI: 10.1007/BF02236694

[25] Pilkington SA, Bhome R, Welch RE, Ku F, Warden C, Harris S, et al. Bilateral versus unilateral botulinum toxin injections for chronic anal fissure: A randomised trial. Techniques in Coloproctology. 2018;**22**(7):545-551. DOI: 10.1007/s10151-018-1821-2

[26] Ravindran P, Chan DL, Ciampa C, George R, Punch G, White SI. High-dose versus low-dose botulinum toxin in anal fissure disease. Techniques in Coloproctology. 2017;**21**(10):803-808. DOI: 10.1007/s10151-017-1700-2

[27] Bobkiewicz A, Francuzik W, Krokowicz L, Studniarek A, Ledwosiński W, Paszkowski J, et al. Botulinum toxin injection for treatment of chronic anal fissure: Is there any dose-dependent efficiency? A meta-analysis. World Journal of Surgery. 2016;**40**(12):3064-3072. DOI: 10.1007/s00268-016-3693-9

[28] Brisinda G, Cadeddu F, Brandara F, Marniga G, Maria G. Randomized clinical trial comparing botulinum toxin injections with 0.2 per cent nitroglycerin ointment for chronic anal fissure. The British Journal of Surgery. 2007;**94**(2):162-167. DOI: 10.1002/bjs.5514

[29] Fruehauf H, Fried M, Wegmueller B, Bauerfeind P, Thumshirn M. Efficacy and safety of botulinum toxin a injection compared with topical nitroglycerin ointment for the treatment of chronic anal fissure: A prospective randomized study. The American Journal of Gastroenterology.

2006;**101**(9):2107-2112. DOI: 10.1111/j.1572-0241.2006.00722.x

[30] De Nardi P, Ortolano E, Radaelli G, Staudacher C. Comparison of glycerine trinitrate and botulinum toxin-a for the treatment of chronic anal fissure: Long-term results. Diseases of the Colon and Rectum. 2006;**49**(4):427-432. DOI: 10.1007/s10350-005-0287-2

[31] Sahebally SM, Meshkat B, Walsh SR, Beddy D. Botulinum toxin injection vs topical nitrates for chronic anal fissure: An updated systematic review and meta-analysis of randomized controlled trials. Colorectal Disease. 2018;**20**(1):6-15. DOI: 10.1111/codi.13969

[32] Samim M, Twigt B, Stoker L, Pronk A. Topical diltiazem cream versus botulinum toxin a for the treatment of chronic anal fissure: A double-blind randomized clinical trial. Annals of Surgery. 2012;**255**:18-22

[33] Sajid MS, Vijaynagar B, Desai M, Cheek E, Baig MK. Botulinum toxin vs glyceryltrinitrate for the medical management of chronic anal fissure: A meta-analysis. Colorectal Disease. 2008;**10**(6):541-546. DOI: 10.1111/j.1463-1318.2007.01387.x

[34] Gil J, Luján J, Hernández Q, Gil E, Salom MG, Parrilla P. Screening for the effectiveness of conservative treatment in chronic anal fissure patients using anorectal manometry. International Journal of Colorectal Disease. 2010;**25**(5): 649-654. DOI: 10.1007/s00384-010-0885-x

[35] Smith M, Frizelle F. Long-term faecal incontinence following the use of botulinum toxin. Colorectal Disease. 2004;**6**(6):526-527. DOI: 10.1111/j.1463-1318.2004.00720.x

[36] Brown SR, Matabudul Y, Shorthouse AJ. A second case of long-term incontinence following botulinum injection for anal fissure. Colorectal Disease. 2006;**8**(5):452-453. DOI: 10.1111/j.1463-1318.2006.00964.x

[37] Bhama AR, Zoccali MB, Chapman BC, Davids JS, Eisenstein S, Fish DR, et al. Practice variations in Chemodenervation for anal fissure among American Society of Colon and Rectal Surgeons members. Diseases of the Colon and Rectum. 2021;**64**(10):1167-1171. DOI: 10.1097/DCR.0000000000002194

[38] Nelson RL, Manuel D, Gumienny C, Spencer B, Patel K, Schmitt K, et al. A systematic review and meta-analysis of the treatment of anal fissure. Techniques in Coloproctology. 2017;**21**(8):605-625. DOI: 10.1007/s10151-017-1664-2

[39] Massoud BW, Mehrdad V, Baharak T, Alireza Z. Botulinum toxin injection versus internal anal sphincterotomy for the treatment of chronic anal fissure. Annals of Saudi Medicine. 2005;**25**: 140-142

[40] Iswariah H, Stephens J, Rieger N, Rodda D, Hewett P. Randomized prospective controlled trial of lateral internal sphincterotomy versus injection of botulinum toxin for the treatment of idiopathic fissure in ano. ANZ Journal of Surgery. 2005;**75**:553-555

[41] Valizadeh N, Jalaly NY, Hassanzadeh M, et al. Botulinum toxin injection versus lateral internal sphincterotomy for the treatment of chronic anal fissure: Randomized prospective controlled trial. Langenbeck's Archives of Surgery. 2012;**397**:1093-1098

[42] Nasr M, Ezzat H, Elsebae M. Botulinum toxin injection versus lateral internal sphincterotomy in the treatment of chronic anal fissure: A randomized controlled trial. World Journal of Surgery. 2010;**34**:2730-2734

[43] Mentes BB, Irko¨rucu O, Akin M, Leventoglu S, Tatlicioglu E. Comparison of botulinum toxin injection and lateral internal sphincterotomy for the treatment of chronic anal fissure. Diseases of the Colon and Rectum. 2003;**46**:232-237

[44] Arroyo Sebastian A, Perez F, Serrano P, Candela F, Lacueva J, Calpena R. Surgical versus chemical (botulinum toxin) sphincterotomy for chronic anal fissure: Long term results of a prospective randomized clinical and manometric study. American Journal of Surgery. 2005;**189**:429-434

[45] Jin JZ, Bhat S, Park B, Hardy MO, Unasa H, Mauiliu-Wallis M, et al. A systematic review and network meta-analysis comparing treatments for anal fissure. Surgery. 2022;**5**:S0039-6060(21)01178-8. DOI: 10.1016/j.surg.2021.11.030

[46] Garg P, Garg M, Menon GR. Long-term continence disturbance after lateral internal sphincterotomy for chronic anal fissure: A systematic review and meta-analysis. Colorectal Disease. 2013;**15**(3):e104-e117. DOI: 10.1111/codi.12108

[47] Menteş BB, Tezcaner T, Yilmaz U, Leventoğlu S, Oguz M. Results of lateral internal sphincterotomy for chronic anal fissure with particular reference to quality of life. Diseases of the Colon and Rectum. 2006;**49**(7):1045-1051. DOI: 10.1007/s10350-006-0527-0

[48] Gupta V, Rodrigues G, Prabhu R, Ravi C. Open versus closed lateral internal anal sphincterotomy in the management of chronic anal fissures: A prospective randomized study. Asian Journal of Surgery. 2014;**37**(4):178-183. DOI: 10.1016/j.asjsur.2014.01.009

[49] Pernkoft BJ, Eisenstat TE, Oliver GC, Salvati EP. Reappraisal of partial lateral internal sphincterotomy. Diseases of the Colon and Rectum. 1994;**7**:1291-1295

[50] Kortbeek JB, Langevin JM, Khoo RE, Heine JA. Chronic fissurein-ano: A randomized study comparing open and subcutaneous lateral internal sphincterotomy. Diseases of the Colon and Rectum. 1992;**35**:835-837

[51] Garcia-Aguilar J, Belmonte C, Wong WD, Lowry AC, Madoff RD. Open vs closed sphincterotomy for chronic anal fissure: Long term results. Diseases of the Colon and Rectum. 1996;**39**:440-443

[52] Altomare DF, Rinaldi M, Troilo VL, Marino F, Lobascio P, Puglisi F. Closed ambulatory lateral internal sphincterotomy for chronic anal fissures. Techniques in Coloproctology. 2005;**9**:248-249

[53] Wiley M, Day P, Rieger N, Stephens J, Moore J. Open vs. closed lateral internal sphincterotomy for idiopathic fissure-in-ano: A prospective, randomized, controlled trial. Diseases of the Colon and Rectum. 2004;**47**(6):847-852. DOI: 10.1007/s10350-004-0530-2

[54] Arroyo A, Pérez F, Serrano P, Candela F, Calpena R. Open versus closed lateral sphincterotomy performed as an outpatient procedure under local anesthesia for chronic anal fissure: Prospective randomized study of clinical and manometric longterm results. Journal of the American College of Surgeons. 2004;**199**(3):361-367. DOI: 10.1016/j.jamcollsurg.2004.04.016

[55] Ersoz F, Arikan S, Sari S, Bektas H, Ozcan O. Type of lateral internal sphincterotomy incision: Parallel or vertical? World Journal of Surgery. 2011;**35**:1137-1141

[56] Kang WH, Lim CH, Choi DH, Shin HK, Lee YC, Jeong SK, et al.

Comparison of skin incisions used for open lateral internal sphincterotomies--radial versus circumferential incisions: A retrospective cohort study. International Journal of Surgery. 2014;**12**(11):1141-1145. DOI: 10.1016/j.ijsu.2014.09.005

[57] Littlejohn DR, Newstead GL. Tailored lateral sphincterotomy for anal fissure. Diseases of the Colon and Rectum. 1997;**40**(12):1439-1442. DOI: 10.1007/BF02070709

[58] Elsebae MM. A study of fecal incontinence in patients with chronic anal fissure: Prospective, randomized, controlled trial of the extent of internal anal sphincter division during lateral sphincterotomy. World Journal of Surgery. 2007;**31**(10):2052-2057. DOI: 10.1007/s00268-007-9177-1

[59] Mentes BB, Ege B, Leventoglu S, Oguz M, Karadag A. Extent of lateral internal sphincterotomy: Up to the dentate line or up to the fissure apex? Diseases of the Colon and Rectum. 2005;**48**:365-370

[60] García-Granero E, Sanahuja A, García-Botello SA, Faiz O, Esclápez P, Espí A, et al. The ideal lateral internal sphincterotomy: Clinical and endosonographic evaluation following open and closed internal anal sphincterotomy. Colorectal Disease. 2009;**11**(5):502-507. DOI: 10.1111/j.1463-1318.2008.01645.x

[61] Murad-Regadas SM, Fernandes GO, Regadas FS, Rodrigues LV, Pereira Jde J, Regadas Filho FS, et al. How much of the internal sphincter may be divided during lateral sphincterotomy for chronic anal fissure in women? Morphologic and functional evaluation after sphincterotomy. Diseases of the Colon and Rectum. 2013;**56**(5):645-651. DOI: 10.1097/DCR.0b013e31827a7416

[62] Brillantino A, Izzo D, Iacobellis F, Maglio M, Grillo M, Vicenzo L, et al. Safety and effectiveness of minimal sphincterotomy in the treatment of female patients with chronic anal fissure. Updates in Surgery. 2021;**73**(5):1829-1836. DOI: 10.1007/s13304-020-00874-8

[63] Sungurtekin U, Ozgen U, Sungurtekin H. Prospective, randomized, controlled trial of ultra-modified internal Sphincterotomy vs closed lateral internal Sphincterotomy for chronic fissure-in-Ano. The American Surgeon. 2021;**16**:31348211011104. DOI: 10.1177/00031348211011104

[64] Cho D-Y. Controlled lateral sphincterotomy for chronic anal fissure. Diseases of the Colon and Rectum. 2004;**48**:1037-1041

[65] Menteş BB, Güner MK, Leventoglu S, Akyürek N. Fine-tuning of the extent of lateral internal sphincterotomy: Spasm-controlled vs. up to the fissure apex. Diseases of the Colon and Rectum. 2008;**51**(1):128-133. DOI: 10.1007/s10350-007-9121-3

Section 2

Hemorrhoids

Chapter 3

Prolapsing Hemorrhoids

Sigit Adi Prasetyo, Parish Budiono and Ignatius Riwanto

Abstract

Hemorrhoids are a common anorectal disease and are often found in clinical practice. Patients mostly come with a complaint of anal bleeding or prolapsing mass. Grade III and IV prolapsing hemorrhoids are distinguished from grade II by the fact that grade II prolapse only during defecation and returns simultaneously after defecation and usually does not cause complaint. Prolapsing hemorrhoids should be differentiated from prolapsing rectal polyps, small rectal prolapse, anorectal tumors, hypertrophy of the anal papilla, and condylomas. Nowadays, the management of prolapsing hemorrhoids varies. Medical therapy is rarely used alone, it is used to improve the effect of surgical therapy. The surgical gold standard for prolapsing hemorrhoids is excision surgery (hemorrhoidectomy) with or without suturing. However, since it comes with pain complaints, non-excision surgery is now offered. Non-excision surgery is divided into two types—stapled hemorrhoidopexy and hemorrhoidal artery ligation and rectoanal repair. Each method of surgery has its own advantages and disadvantages. This chapter review discusses the anatomy, pathophysiology, diagnosis, and management of prolapsing hemorrhoids.

Keywords: hemorrhoids prolapse, hemorrhoidectomy, hemorrhoidopexy

1. Introduction

Hemorrhoids are a disease of the anorectal area, that is often found in clinical practice, it is an enlargement and prolapsing (shift to the distal) of the anal cushion that gives clinical signs and symptoms [1]. Dilation and deformity of the blood vessels in the anal cushions, accompanied by destruction of the supporting tissues are the main pathological conditions of hemorrhoids. Inflammatory reactions and hyperplasia of blood vessels can also be found in hemorrhoids [2, 3].

Patients with complaints of bloody stools or anal discomfort are often caused by hemorrhoids, but the exact prevalence is unknown and will be lower than reality because many are under-reported and patients are self-medicating. The prevalence varies greatly from country to country, depending on the recording system. Data in the United States in 1990 showed that more than 10 million people suffered from hemorrhoids, or about 4.4% of the total population, while in the UK it was reported to be 13–36% of the general population [3]. The prevalence of men and women is comparable, and mostly occurs at the age of 45–65 years. White and high socioeconomic populations are more frequently affected than blacks and low socioeconomic populations [2].

Considering that hemorrhoids are the most common anal canal abnormalities and also the reason for patients' visits to the doctor or physician, a deep understanding of the anatomy, physiology, pathogenesis, risk factors, diagnosis, and rational management is needed for doctors, to be able to treat hemorrhoids correctly and effectively, so that the patient is protected from irresponsible hemorrhoid management practices.

2. Anatomy and physiology

The anal canal is a continuation of the distal rectum. The surgical anal canal is formed by the hindgut in the proximal part and the anoderm in the distal part, and the border between both is dentate lines. The proximal part of the anus is covered by a mucous line. The superior rectal artery that flows through the anal canal will branch into two, to the left and right. The right branch of the superior rectal artery branches into anterior and posterior branches. This artery will form an arteriovenous plexus located in the right anterior, right posterior, and left lateral regions, which will be covered by mucosa that produces an anal cushion. For practical purposes, from a perineal view, we call it 11.00 o'clock the right anterior, 07.00 o'clock the right posterior, and 03.00 o'clock the left lateral anal cushion [4].

There are two anal canal sphincters, the internal anal canal sphincter (IAS) as a continuation and thickening of the circular layer of rectal muscle and the external anal sphincter (EAS). The IAS is made of smooth muscle. It is an involutory muscle, while the external sphincter muscle is a voluntary muscle consisting of three layers—deep, superficial, and subcutaneous [1]. Anal incontinence during rest is caused by the contraction of the IAS and anal cushion, which participate 70–80% and 20–30%, respectively. During defecation, the anal cushion will prolapse downward to protect the anal crypt, estuary of the anal gland, and anal canal skin, and return after defecation. The ability of the anal cushion to return is due to the function of the muscle of Treitz, the continuation of muscle fiber from the longitudinal muscle fiber of the rectum. The Treitz muscle consists of two parts—the submucous muscle and the Park ligament, where the last part of it is located at the bottom of the anal cushion [4].

According to Aigner, et al., (2009), there are sphincter-like structures in the vascular plexus, formed by thickened tunica media that contain 5–15 layers of smooth muscle cells located between the vascular plexus and the subepithelial space of the anal cushions in normal anorectal specimens. The role of these sphincter-like structures is to coordinate the filling and drainage of the anorectal vascular plexus. This vascular plexus is without tunica media and larger than usual, like a lacuna [5].

3. Pathogenesis and risk factors

The pathogenesis of hemorrhoids is still largely unknown. Hemorrhoids occur based on the theory of varicose veins, as in the case of leg varicose veins, but in the case of hemorrhoids, they occur in the anus. This theory has been abandoned because various studies have shown that varicose veins and hemorrhoids are different entities. There was no increase in the incidence of hemorrhoids in patients with portal hypertension. The theories of vascular hyperplasia and hypertrophy of the anal sphincter are not supported by the evidence. Today, the theory of the sliding of the anal cushions is widely accepted [2, 4].

As it has been stated in the physiology of the anus and rectum, the anal cushion plays a role in protecting the anal canal during defecation. After the stool comes out, the anus cushions will return to their place due to the work of the Treitz muscles.

In constipation, there will be difficulty in defecating. The patient will push a lot so that the anal cushions are often forced to shift distally. Over time, it will be followed by damage to the supporting tissue, so that the anal cushions cannot return to their own position. Prolapsing anal cushions will be followed by venous dilatation, vascular thrombosis, degeneration of fibroelastic tissue, and damage to the Treitz muscles. Inflammatory reactions are also seen in the vascular wall and the surrounding supporting tissues, ulceration, ischemia, and thrombosis [4].

Several enzymes play a role in the degradation of the supporting tissues of the anal pads. Matrix metalloproteinase (MMP), a zinc-dependent proteinase, is the most potent enzyme and is capable of degrading elastin, fibronectin, and collagen. MMP-9 is overexpressed in hemorrhoids and degrades elastin fibers. Activation of MMP-2 and MMP-9 by thrombin, plasmin or other proteinases results in damage to the capillary bed and stimulates the vascular proliferative activity of TGF (transforming growth factor). This also explains the thinning of the tunica media in the sphincter-like structures that control blood flow from the arteries to the venous plexus. Hemorrhoids have an overexpressed endoglin attachment site with TGF. Microvascular density also increases, influenced by Vascular Endothelial Growth Factors (VEGF), which increases, especially when there is thrombosis [4].

Morphological and hemodynamic studies showed that in hemorrhoids there was an increase in the diameter of the branches of the superior rectal artery, the amount of blood flowing and its flow rate increased significantly. There is a correlation between the diameter of the arterial branches and the degree of hemorrhoids [6]. Physiological changes in the anal canal in hemorrhoids have also been reported. Anal canal pressure at rest in patients with prolapsed and unprolapsed hemorrhoids was higher than in normal people, without internal anal sphincter hypertrophy. This pressure will decrease after hemorrhoidectomy is performed, so it can be said that this increase in pressure is due to the effect of hemorrhoids, not the cause [7].

Constipation is widely believed to be a risk factor for the occurrence of hemorrhoids, through the sliding mechanism of the anal cushion, as previously stated, but diarrhea has also been reported to increase the risk of hemorrhoids, through an unclear mechanism. Pregnancy is also a predisposing factor for hemorrhoids due to increased intra-abdominal pressure causing congestion of the anal cushion, and the patient can recover after delivery. Many other risk factors have been reported for the occurrence of hemorrhoids, such as a low-fiber diet, spicy foods, and drinking alcohol [2, 4, 7].

4. Pathology and grading

Hemorrhoids due to prolapse of the anal cushions are called internal hemorrhoids. The lump is covered with mucosa and is often accompanied by the skin of the anal canal, thus forming mixed hemorrhoids, but the predominance is internal hemorrhoids. If only the external hemorrhoidal plexus is dilated, it is called external hemorrhoids. On histological examination of the surgical specimen for internal hemorrhoids, a very marked widening of the vascular plexus and fragmentation of the Treitz muscles will be found. When examined deeply, an increase in leukocytes both inside and outside the blood vessels (inflammatory component) and, with special staining, thinning of the blood vessel walls due to thinning of the tunica media (sphincter-forming muscles) will be seen. External hemorrhoids are mainly dilated subcutaneous veins accompanied by an inflammatory reaction, but patients often present with pain due to a thrombus [2–4].

Stages of internal hemorrhoids need to be determined before starting therapy because the stage will greatly determine the choice of therapy. **Goligher** was the expert who first proposed the degree of hemorrhoids, so the Goligher classification is known, and is still used today (**Figure 1**) [8].

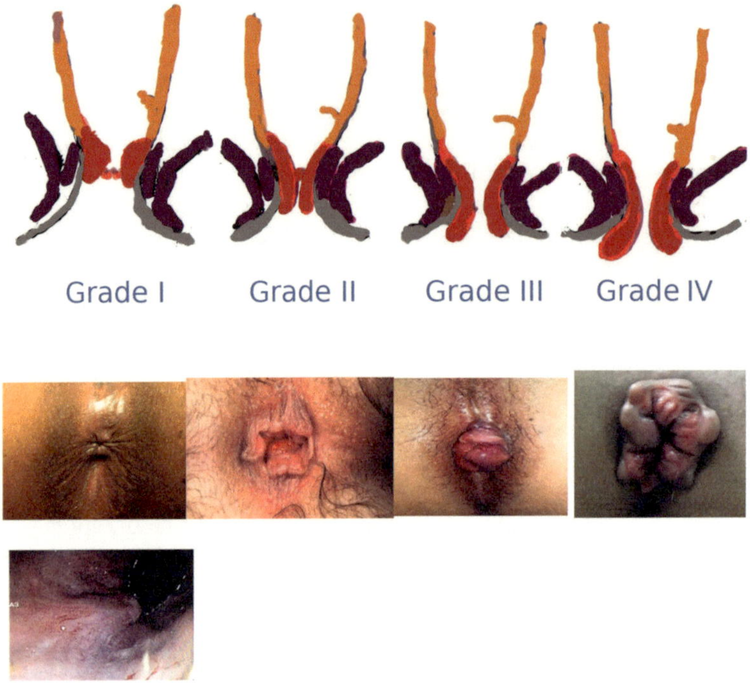

Figure 1.
Internal Hemorrhoid grade. Grade I: no prolapse seen from outside, but can be seen by u-turn colonoscopy, Grade II: the lump can be seen during straining and spontaneously return after straining is completed. Grade III: the lump can be seen during and after straining and only by manual help can be reduced to its positions. Grade IV: The lump is already outside the anus, and cannot or fail to be reduced.

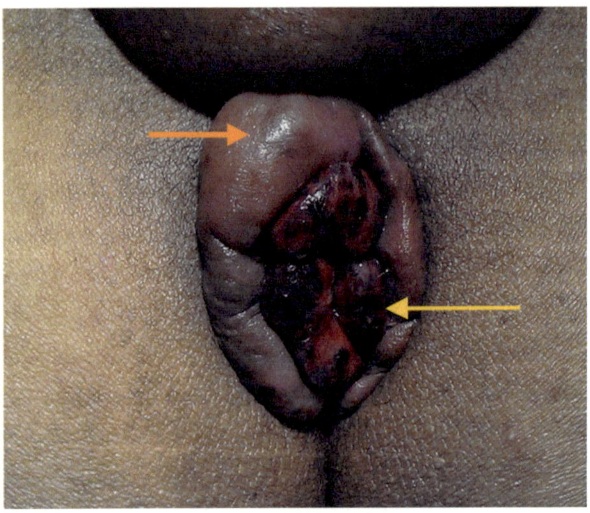

Figure 2.
Grade IV mixed hemorrhoids with thrombus in external (orange arrow) and internal (yellow arrow) components.

Grade I: anal cushion bleeding but no prolapse. Grade II: anal cushions prolapse out of the anus during defecation, but can spontaneously return. Grade III: prolapsed anal cushions that protrude from the anus during defecation but require manual assistance to return to their original position. Grade IV: prolapsed anal cushions out the anus and cannot be reposed manually.

The American Society of Colorectal Surgery (ASCS) made a modification to Goligher grading because in Goligher the classification is based on what the patient says, but in ASCS it is based more on examination. In grades II and III, a Valsalva test should be performed, while in grade IV, this includes being able to manually reposition the prolapsed anal cushions, which will soon come back out. In grade IV, due to obstruction of venous return by the anal sphincter, often accompanied by incarceration and thrombosis under the anal mucosa or skin (**Figure 2**).

5. Diagnosis

5.1 Differential diagnosis

Because patients often present with fresh bloody stools and lumps in the anus, the following diseases should be considered: Anorectal malignancy (adenocarcinoma, squamous cell carcinoma, and malignant melanoma), rectal prolapse, prolapsed rectal polyp, anal fistula, anal fissure, Crohn's disease, and condyloma acuminata [2]. Each has different signs and symptoms, so recognizing the signs and symptoms of each will lead to a good diagnosis.

5.2 Signs and symptoms

Bleeding in hemorrhoids is often fresh red blood without pain. This is different from an acute anal fissure, which causes fresh bloody stools accompanied by intense pain because there is an injury in the anal canal skin, which is rich in pain receptor nerves (somatic nerves). The color of the blood in hemorrhoidal bleeding is fresh because the source of the blood is the arteriovenous shunt. Rectal bleeding in rectal carcinoma is often reddish, along with the mucus. Left colon carcinoma is often accompanied by small stools with blood on their surface, while bleeding in the right colon carcinoma is often brown in color with diarrhea. A positive occult blood test should be considered more proximal to the source of bleeding, so a colonoscopy is recommended to detect the source of bleeding [1]. The prolapsed mucosa will secrete mucus which can irritate the anal skin, causing itching. In large hemorrhoids, the patient may feel incomplete defecation or feeling of fullness in the rectum. Pain in hemorrhoids only occurs when a thrombus occurs, especially in the blood vessels under the skin or at grade IV, which is constricted by a strong anal sphincter, causing strangulation [3].

5.3 Physical examination

With the patient in the lithotomy or Sim's position, laying on the left side with maximum flexion in the hip and knee joints, inspections are carried out in the perineal and anal areas to detect possible skin tags, external hemorrhoids, skin inflammation due to irritation by mucus and feces, the presence of fissures or anal fistula. (**Figure 3**). When the prolapsed anal cushion is visible, it is necessary to identify the position and number of the main lumps, the presence or absence of the prolapsed anal canal skin, and the presence of thrombus or ulceration [3].

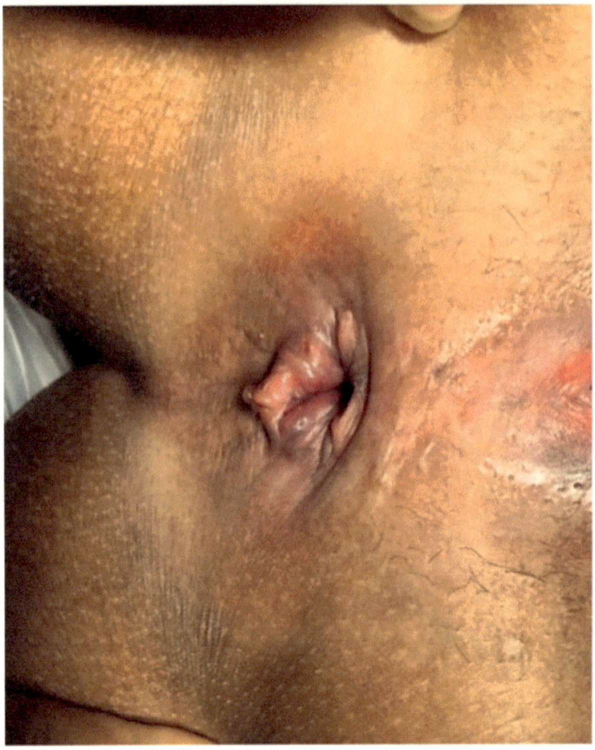

Figure 3.
In Sim's position, spreading the anus by the left and right finger and asking the patient to strain, two nodules can be seen at 03.00, and 07.00 o'clock, in this case, anal fissure can also be seen at 06.00 o;clock (black arrow). (Personal collection).

Keep in mind that, other than hemorrhoids, other prolapses are rectal prolapse and rectal polyps. In a prolapsed rectal polyp, it will appear as a round lump covered with mucosa and have a stalk (**Figure 4a** and **b**). The rectal prolapse is concentric or circular in shape (not lumpy or no radial indentation), not followed by prolapse of the anal skin, and the finger can enter between the prolapse and the anal canal wall [9]. If during the initial examination there is no prolapsed lump, the patient is asked to strain so that prolapse can occur, or more effectively, the patient is asked to squat and be asked to push into the toilet. In addition to the prolapse examination as mentioned above, wait a while to observe the ability of the prolapsing anal cushion to spontaneously disappear, due to self repositioning, or must be pushed with your fingers [8].

Anal melanoma can affect the anal canal and distal rectum, and the majority of tumors are located within 6 cm proximal to the anal verge. There are two types, melanotic, which consists 70% of cases and amelanotic 30%. Amelanotic melanoma is mostly located in the mucosa. Anal melanoma is a rare anal neoplasm. It accounts for approximately 1–4% of anal neoplasms and is female predominant. The signs are an anal lump, pain, and bleeding [10].

Melanotic anal melanoma can be confused with hemorrhoids with thrombosis, as both cause black discoloration. Hemorrhoid thrombus is usually more painful, and the pain will subside after day 3 due to the shrinkage of the lump. This phenomenon is not found in melanotic anal melanoma. The presence of a satellite nodule is also specific to melanoma (**Figure 5a**). The diagnosis is based on the histological picture

DOI: http://dx.doi.org/10.5772/intechopen.104554

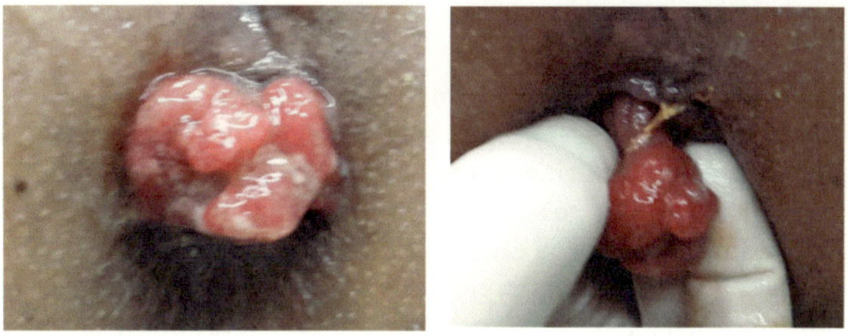

a b

Figure 4.
a. Prolapse of rectal polyps, b. the polyps stalk can be seen after retracted outside. (Personal collection).

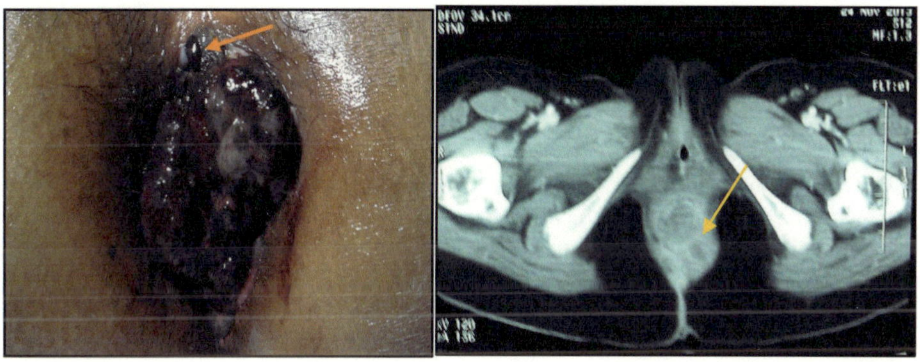

(a) (b)

Figure 5.
Anal melanoma, melanotic type. a. with satellite nodule (arrow), b. infiltration to anal sphincter on CT scan (Personal collection).

of the biopsy specimen. A CT scan is needed to confirm the degree of infiltration, lymph node involvement, and distant metastasis. In **Figure 5b**, the tumor has already infiltrated the anal sphincter. The abdominal perineal ano-recto-sigmoidectomy (Mile's procedure) with permanent sigmoidostomy is the surgery of choice [1, 10].

The patient should also have a digital rectal examination (DRE). Uncomplicated internal hemorrhoids are often vaguely palpable as a soft anorectal mass that is absent in normal people, but when a thrombus or scar tissue has occurred, something harder or a narrowing due to a stricture may be felt. During DRE, anal sphincter tone, prostate enlargement, and the presence of other abnormalities in the rectum, as well as outside the rectum in women, such as the uterus and adnexa, should also be evaluated. To palpate rectal cancer that cannot be reached by fingers, it can be done bimanually (one hand on the lower abdomen and pressing down) or the patient is asked to push (Valsalva test). When there is a rectal tumor in a high position and mobile, it is often palpable with the maximal position of the finger during a digital rectal examination. Patients with complaints of pain in the rectal area have the possibility of fissures, but there is also the possibility of arthritis of the sacro-coccigeal joint. For this reason, during a digital rectal examination, it should not be forgotten to move the coccyx from the sacrum bone. The presence of arthritis will cause pain with movement [1, 3].

5.4 Endoscopy

During anuscopy, the size of the hemorrhoidal nodule, position, level of inflammation, and the possibility of bleeding should be assessed. When a colonoscopy is performed, the retroflexed position of the scope can see hemorrhoids in the rectum. Likewise, a transparent anoscope can clearly see the anal canal and hemorrhoids. Photo documentation can be made during endoscopy [1–3].

As rectal bleeding is the main complaint of internal hemorrhoid, should a routine complete colon examination be done to rule out other causes of bleeding? American Society of Colon and Rectal Surgeons (ASRC) recommends patients with—a) rectal bleeding, b) positive fecal immunochemical testing (FTT), c) positive FTT-fecal DNA test, d) patients with high risk for colorectal malignancy such as d.1) age 50 years or more if no complete examination within 10 years, d.2) age 40 years or more or 10 years younger with history of first degree relative of colorectal cancer or advanced adenoma diagnosed at age less than 60 years, and d.3) age 40 years or more or 10 years younger with history positive for two first degree relatives with advance adenomas or colorectal carcinomas [8].

5.5 Complications

The most common complication for hemorrhoid patients is bleeding. Bleeding varies, from just spots that drip after defecation to heavy bleeding chronic. Slight bleeding may result in microcytic hypochromic anemia, while if the bleeding is profuse, patients may come down with hypovolemic shock. The profuse bleeding is an emergency, so it must be managed immediately [1–3]. Another complication is thrombosis of the veins, which can be located under the mucosa or the skin. Thrombosis of the skin or mucosa near the skin will be very painful, prompting the patient to seek treatment immediately. Prolapsed hemorrhoids accompanied by a strong anal sphincter can result in compression of the blood flow, resulting in strangulation and even necrosis [1].

5.6 Management

Management of hemorrhoids depends on the stage. Management includes dietetic management and lifestyle changes (controlling risk factors), administration of drugs, and nonsurgical and surgical interventions. In grade I, II, and small III hemorrhoids, management starts with dietetic management, changing lifestyle, and administration of drugs, if those fail then nonsurgical intervention is considered. In major stages III and IV, the main choice is surgery plus dietetic management and lifestyle changes. In cases of acute thrombosis or strangulation, emergency surgery is required [8].

5.7 Dietetic management and lifestyle modifications

Patients with hemorrhoids are very prone to bleeding, and the lumps may become more swollen when the stool is hard because the defecation must be strained hard. To avoid this, the stool must be soft so that it does not cause trauma. This could be achieved by increasing a high-fiber diet or adding a bulking laxative to the diet, such as bran or methylcellulose, to facilitate defecation. A meta-analysis study showed that a high-fiber diet reduced the risk of complaints and bleeding in up to 50% of cases, although it did not improve complaints of prolapse, pain, and itching [11]. A high-fiber diet is very effective for hemorrhoids that do not prolapse [1, 3].

Controlling the manageable risk factors by modification of lifestyle plays a role in the healing process of hemorrhoids [3]. Patients who initially do not like fiber foods should be advised to consume high fiber, drink enough water, and do regular physical activity to facilitate defecation. The recommended amount of fiber per day is 35 gr [1]. Foods that contain high fat should be avoided because they do not support the formation of large and loose stools, as well as drugs that cause constipation or even diarrhea, should also be avoided. The wrong way of defecating must be corrected. Avoid defecating by pushing too hard and sitting on the toilet for too long (smoking, reading newspapers, playing with cell phones, etc.) [2]. By squatting, it is easier to pass stool, because the puborectal muscle is more relaxed. One study shows that defecating in a squatting position only takes 1 minute, as opposed to a sitting position that needs 4–15 minutes [12]. When you are used to defecating by sitting on the toilet, by propping your feet higher, the position would be more like squatting. After defecation, the anoperineal must be clean. Remaining feces in the anal canal, for example in the anal crypts, can stimulate inflammation.

6. Medicamentous treatment

6.1 Flavonoids

Flavonoids are herbal medicines that are given orally. This drug was originally indicated as a blood vessel strengthening agent (venotonic) and an anti-edema agent in the treatment of varicose veins in the legs. These flavonoids have been studied in varicose veins. They have the ability to increase vascular tone, decrease venous capacity, decrease capillary permeability, increase lymphatic drainage, and have anti-inflammatory effects. Although the mechanism of healing in hemorrhoids is not clear, this drug has been widely used in Europe and Asia. The micronized purified flavonoid fraction (MPFF) consisting of 90% diosmin and 10% hesperidin is the most commonly used flavonoid in clinical practice. This fine shape (less than 2 microns in size), allows absorption to be easier so that it works faster [13].

A recent meta-analysis showed that MPFF treatment provided significant benefits for bleeding (odds ratio [OR] 0.082, $p < 0.001$), discharge/leakage (OR 0.12, $p < 0.001$), and overall improvement according to patients (OR 5.25, $p < 0.001$) and investigators (OR 5.51, $p < 0.001$). MPFF also reduces pain (OR 0.11, $P = 0.06$) [14]. The recommended dose in the acute phase is 3x1 gr in the first 3–4 days and then decreases to 2x1 gr. The medication can be stopped gradually, according to the patient's response. Long-term use of this medication is reported to be safe. The medication is also reported to be safe to be used in pregnant women [13].

Purple leaf (Grapthopylum pictum extract/GPE), which also contains flavonoids, has been shown to be useful in improving the complaints of hemorrhoids in developing countries. In a study for patients with hemorrhoids, with a pre and post-test-only group design, it was reported that GPE reduces the signs and symptoms [15]. In animal studies, inducing anal Wistar rats with croton oil, showed that GPE, reduces inflammatory markers [16], accelerates ulcer healing [17], and reduces edema [18]. Currently, in Indonesia, GPE can be considered a standardized herb. To be recognized as a phytopharmaca, it needs to be continued with better clinical trials.

6.2 Calcium dobesilate

It is an oral drug that has a venotonic effect (strengthens veins), reduces capillary permeability, inhibits thrombotic aggregation, and increases blood viscosity, which results in reducing edema. Calcium dobesilates are often used for leg varicose veins and diabetic retinopathy. Research on hemorrhoids using calcium dobesilate combined with fiber supplementation has also shown good clinical effects, namely reducing bleeding and inflammation [2].

6.3 Topical treatment

Forms of topical treatment of hemorrhoids are zalf, cream, or rectal suppositories. The purpose of topical treatment is to reduce the symptoms, so most of the ingredients are local anesthetics, corticosteroids, antibiotics, and anti-inflammatory drugs. There is not yet sufficient scientific evidence to support the use of topical treatment [8]. This drug can be purchased without a prescription. It is important to remember that topical treatments are only used in the acute stage. Long-term use of topical treatment can result in thinning the mucosa so that it bleeds easily or the possibility of fungal growth. It is highly recommended that after the acute stage has passed, the drug should be stopped and other drugs given orally, such as the flavonoids described above, should be continued zalf containing 0.2% glyceryl trinitrate or nifedipine, a calcium channel blocker, has been reported to reduce pain due to relaxation of the internal anal sphincter. There is also a topical vasoconstrictor, namely zalf, which contains 0.25% phenylephrine and is reported to reduce the complaints of hemorrhoid patients [19].

6.4 Instrumentation

In the early stages of hemorrhoids, instrumentation can be performed in the private practice room, so it is called an "office-based procedure." External hemorrhoids with thrombus—the thrombus can be removed under local anesthesia, while internal hemorrhoids can be performed with instrumentation. There are various types of instrumentation therapy, but the principle of action is the same. By performing fibrotization at the base of hemorrhoid, it is expected that the blood flow to the anal cushion will decrease and the prolapsed anal cushion will be shrunk and attracted cranially [2, 3].

6.5 Thrombectomy

Thrombectomy is the procedure of removing a thrombus (blood clot) from external hemorrhoid with a thrombus, performed under local anesthesia (**Figure 6a**). The pain of external hemorrhoids with thrombus occurs on the first day, and after the third day, the pain will decrease. Removing the thrombus will quickly relieve the pain. After the 3rd day, because the pain has subsided, there is no indication of thrombectomy. External hemorrhoid will heal through fibrotization of the thrombus into a skin tag [20].

6.6 Sclerotherapy

Submucosal injection at the base of hemorrhoid (**Figure 6b**) with sclerosing agents, such as 5% phenol in oil, vegetable oil, quinine, urea hydrochloride, and hypertonic saline, will result in fibrotization at the base of hemorrhoid so that the

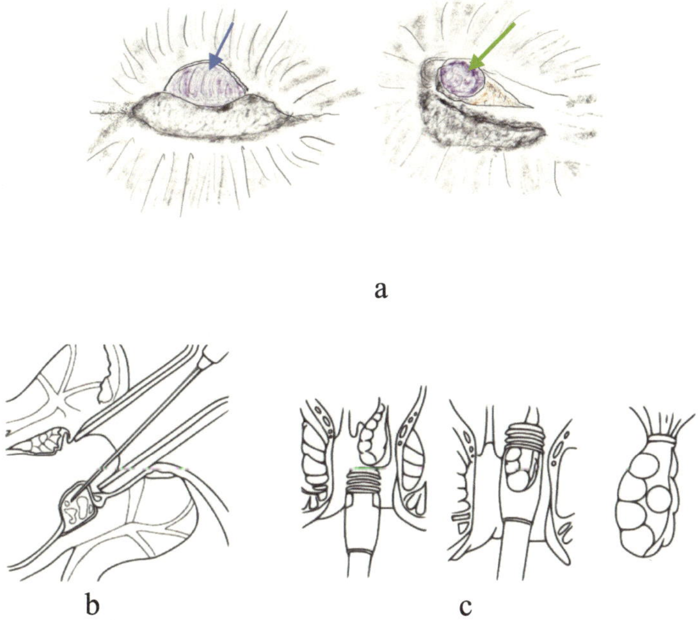

Figure 6.
Office-based procedure a. External hemorrhoid with thrombus, before and after excision b. Sclerotherapy c. Rubber Band Ligation. (illustrated by Kanaya).

anal cushion will be retracted cranially. Injections are often needed several times until the anal cushion is in a normal position. Sclerotherapy is indicated in grade I, and II hemorrhoids [3]. The correct injection should be perivasal. Injection errors may cause problems. Too superficially, they may cause ulceration. Too deep into the muscle causes pain and possibly strictures. Injections into the plexus venosus can cause upper abdominal or precordial pain. Too deep into the prostate can result in an abscess and damage the periprostatic nerves, which can cause erectile dysfunction. Or it can be as serious as retroperitoneal sepsis, as reported by Barwell et al. (1999) [21]. Prophylactic antibiotics are not needed for sclerotherapy, except for cases with immunodeficiency [1–3].

6.7 Rubber band ligation (RBL)

Binding of hemorrhoids with rubber rings (**Figure 6c**) will result in ischemia, necrosis, and healing by the formation of scar tissue that will fix the remaining connective tissue to the rectal wall. RBL is indicated for grade I, II, or small grade III hemorrhoids that do not improve with non-interventional treatment. It is important to keep in mind not to do the ligation too close to the dentate line because it will cause severe pain. Research shows ligation at 2 or 3 places at once or sequentially gives the same results, but post-procedural pain is higher in multiple banding [3]. Discomfort or pain in the rectum can be reduced by taking warm baths and avoiding hard stools by consuming high-fiber foods and drinking enough water, or, if necessary, laxatives. Other than pain, complications after RBL include the possibility of bleeding, mucosal ulceration, thrombosis of external hemorrhoids, and, very rarely, pelvic abscess [1, 2].

6.8 Infrared coagulation

An infrared light probe affixed to the base of hemorrhoid through the anoscope for 1.0–1.5 seconds will have an impact on tissue coagulation and evaporation of fluid in the cells so that hemorrhoid will shrink. The necrotic tissue will appear as white spots, which will heal as fibrotic tissue. This technique is safer than sclerotherapy [1].

6.9 Radiofrequency ablation (RFA)

This technique is relatively new, with an RFA spherical electrode anoscope connected to a radiofrequency generator, attached to the hemorrhoid tissue, which causes evaporation and coagulation of the tissue. In this way, the vascular component will be reduced and fixed to the underlying tissue through fibrotic tissue. Complications that have been reported are thrombosis, wound infection, and urinary retention. From the evaluation of this method, the risk of rebleeding and prolapse is still quite high [2].

6.10 Cryotherapy

Freezing hemorrhoid tissue with a cryotherapy probe is claimed to provide low pain because it is carried out at a low temperature, but in fact, several clinical trials have shown prolonged pain, prolapse, and foul-smelling discharge, so this method is now rarely used [2].

6.11 Laser hemorrhoidoplasty

Laser energy can coagulate the venous plexus tissue. The patient is set in the lithotomy position. Local anesthetic infiltration is performed with xylocaine 20 mL 1% around the anal and perianal skin. A C-shape anoscope is used. A small cut is made in the skin of the anal canal close to hemorrhoid to be targeted for the laser shot. Then a small tube is inserted through which the laser probe will pass, followed by laser shots in several places, generally 5-6 shots, but it can be more, depending on the size of hemorrhoid. The direction of the probe and laser beam can be seen in **Figure 7**. After finishing one point, you can move to another point. The results and the complications were not significantly different from Milligan-Morgan hemorrhoidectomy, or stapler, but less painful [22].

Are there any different indications between sclerotherapy and RBL? There is no difference in terms of indication, but RBL can be done for small IIIrd-degree internal hemorrhoids. If there are no different indications, which one is the best? Research comparing sclerotherapy and RBL concluded that RBL is superior in the resolution of anal protrusion but with higher pain [23]. A survey in the Netherlands reported that most surgeons who treat hemorrhoids choose RBL for the first treatment of Grade II or III internal hemorrhoids [24]. A combination of sclerotherapy and RBL can be done and may improve the result. Research by Kanellos et al. (2003) reported that for the treatment of IInd degree hemorrhoids, the combination of sclerotherapy and RBL is significantly more efficient than sclerotherapy or RBL alone, and RBL is better than sclerotherapy [25]. The results of laser hemorrhoidoplasty are promising [22]. But we are still waiting for long-term results in many cases, and the other problem is that the cost is very expensive.

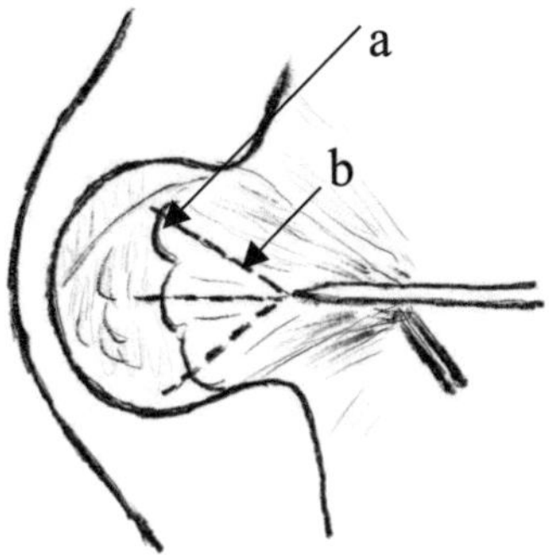

Figure 7.
Laser hemorrhoidoplasty. a. Dentate line, b. Schematic direction of laser shot. (Illustrated by Kanaya).

6.12 Surgical management

Surgical treatment is indicated when nonsurgical treatment is unsuccessful or in hemorrhoids with complications. The presence of strangulation, bleeding that does not stop nonsurgically, and thrombosis indicates emergency surgery. If the presence of other anal canal diseases associated with hemorrhoids, such as fissures and fistulas that require surgery, can be considered for hemorrhoid surgery at once if hemorrhoids are also a complaint [3]. However, surgery is indicated for hemorrhoids in grades III and IV. In general, there are two kinds of surgery—the first is excision of the enlarged and prolapsed anal cushion, and the second is surgery to spare and fix the anal cushion ("anal cushion preserving surgery").

Based on the understanding of the pathogenesis of hemorrhoids as varicose veins, an excision is an option, but based on the theory of sliding or prolapsing of the anal cushion, surgery by fixing the anal cushion toward the cranially is the superior choice. The discovery of increasing caliber and flow of the rectal artery in hemorrhoids and the presence of a sphincter-like structure, in the form of thickening of the tunica media, at the arteriovenous connection, that is thinning or missing in hemorrhoids, [5, 6] superior rectal artery ligation is more rational.

6.13 Excisional hemorrhoidectomy (EH)

EH is a hemorrhoid surgery by removing the hemorrhoids, where nowadays the gold standard is radially removing the three largest lumps (11, 3, and 7 o'clock). Tissues are removed, including the mucosa and the venous plexus below it, without damaging the internal anal sphincter, and maintaining a normal mucosal bridge in between them. After excision, the lump can be left unstitched (Morgan Milligan technique **Figure 8a**) or sutured (Fergusson technique, **Figure 8b**) [1].

It is still debatable which one is better, left open or sewn, because, from various studies, the results are inconsistent. Rationally, in sutured cases, it is very often that the wound will also open in the next couple of days, either because the thread is broken or the tissue is cut. For those reasons, many surgeons choose the open technique. However, a meta-analysis done by Batti et al. (2016) showed the superiority of closed hemorrhoidectomy (Ferguson) over open hemorrhoidectomy (Morgan Milligan) in reducing postoperative pain, risk of postoperative bleeding, and faster wound healing. The only advantage of Morgan Milligan is shorter operative time, while the other

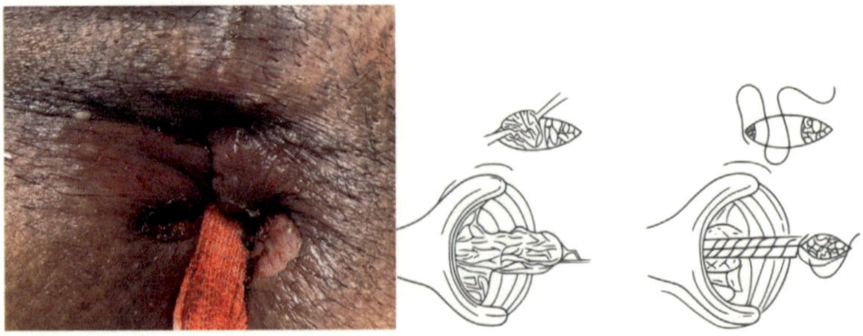

a b

Figure 8.
a. After removing three piles and leaving no suture (Milligan-Morgan) (Personal collection). b. After removing 3 piles and suturing is performed (Ferguson technique) (Illustrated by Kanaya).

aspects, such as length of hospital stay, postoperative complications, recurrence, and risk of surgical site infection, were similar in both groups [26].

There is a circular hemorrhoid excision technique that involves removing the entire lump, including the skin, mucosa, and the underlying venous plexus while maintaining the internal anal sphincter, followed by circular suturing of the skin with the mucosa as well. This technique, known as the Whitehead technique, has been abandoned because of the severe postoperative pain and complications that often arise, namely the risk of injury to the internal anal sphincter, which will cause incontinence, strictures that will cause difficulty passing stools, and exposing the mucosa, which will cause frequent anal canals to be wet (wet anal syndrome/whipping anus) [27]. Because the anal mucosa is rich in nerves and is able to feel and distinguish the desire to defecate solid, liquid, or fart, there are two cases, which I noticed from my personal cases, of patients complaining of the urge to fart but passing stool after Whitehead hemorrhoid surgery. The other method of hemorrhoidectomy technique is submucosal hemorrhoidectomy, which involves removing the venous plexus only (Park's technique). It is currently being discontinued because the technique is more difficult and the risk of bleeding is high [2].

As excisional hemorrhoidectomy is done by removing the anal cushion, the possibility of reducing anal resting pressure after surgery is possible. According to the findings of a study conducted by Li et al. (2012), patients with preoperative compromised continence may have further deterioration of their continence, and thus Milligan-Morgan hemorrhoidectomy should be avoided in such patients [28].

Although the long-term recurrence rate is significantly lower than other methods, the main problem with excisional hemorrhoidectomy is the excruciating postoperative pain. The pain is thought to be caused by a side-burning wound caused by the use of electrocautery. Research shows that the use of lower-temperature cutting energies, such as ligasures or ultrasonic blades (Harmonic scalpel) provides significantly less pain than electrocautery [29].

6.14 Repositioning the anal cushions

The pathology of grade III and IV internal hemorrhoids shows damage to the structure of the supporting tissue of the anal cushions, namely the Treitz muscle and the muscularis mucosae so that if it prolapses, it cannot be repositioned spontaneously but must be repositioned with fingers or cannot be reposed manually. In the beginning, the first effort to treat prolapse is made by performing sutures to fix anal cushions to the base of the hemorrhoids. However, this method still causes problems, namely bleeding and annoying pain, so this method is less attractive [2].

6.14.1 The stapled hemorrhoidopexy (SH)

SH, which was introduced in 1988, is the most widely used method of repositioning the anal cushion [1]. A circular stapler is used to perform a circular excision of the mucosa of the distal rectum and reattach the cut with the stapler, repositioning the prolapsed anal cushions (**Figure 9**).

With circular rectal excision, it is expected that the branch of the superior rectal artery could be cut, and this would result in decreased anal cushion bleeding and the lump would shrink. However, the cutting of the rectal artery cannot be fully realized, because it will depend on the depth of the suture and the location of the artery at the suture level. The research showed that the superior rectal artery was located in the submucosa at 100% at 1 cm above the anorectal ring and 96.6% at 2 cm and 67.1% at 3 cm above the anorectal ring [30]. A study is needed to confirm rectal branch artery cutting in the rectal specimen of stapler hemorrhoidopexy.

A meta-analysis of a randomized controlled trial showed that compared to excisional hemorrhoidectomy, SH provides less pain, a shorter length of stay, and a quicker return to work, but higher long-term recurrence [31, 32]. If the purse-string suture is too deep, it can get into the rectal muscle, which can lead to serious complications. There have been reports of rectovaginal fistulas, pelvic abscesses, and even peritonitis and strictures [2].

6.14.2 Doppler-Guided Hemorrhoid Artery Ligation (DG-HAL)

DG-HAL, developed by Morinaga (Japan) in 1995, is to perform ligation of the distal branch of the superior rectal artery with the help of Doppler to detect the location of the artery so that the ligation will be accurate. From empirical experience, the hemorrhoids will shrink at 6 weeks' follow-up.

Initial experience showed that for grade III and IV hemorrhoids, this procedure did not give satisfactory results, the recurrent rate was still high, so in 2005, the

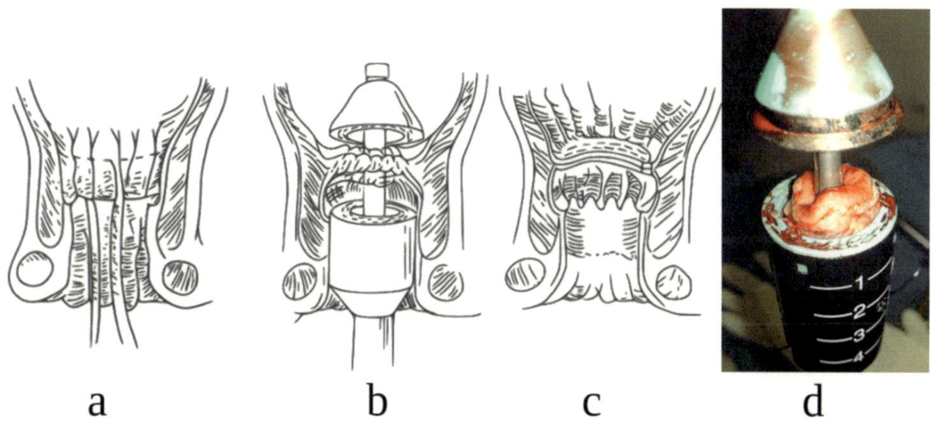

Figure 9.
Stapler hemorrhoidopexy. a. purse-string suture on Morgani column in upper margin of internal hemorrhoids, b. thread knotted between anvil and stapler head, approximate both until save the position and then fire. c.After removing the stapler, the rest of the anal cushion retracted upside, (Illustrated by Kanaya) d. Accurate stapling if we have complete circular rectal tissue like donuts. (personal collection).

DG-HAL procedure was added with rectoanal repair (RAR), (**Figure 10**), namely, performing continuous sutures to fix the anal cushion proximally. To make sure that the anal cushion can move and be fixed proximally, the first stitch in the proximal part should include the rectal muscle and then submucosally. To avoid severe pain, the last suture to fix the anal cushions should be placed above 1 cm from the dentate line [33]. **Figure 11a** and **b** show hemorrhoids before and after DG-HAL-RAR.

The small meta-analysis of 3 RCT, by comparing 70 SH with 80 DG-HAL-RAR, the baseline homogenous (P = 0.40), showed no difference regarding success rate (p = 0.19), operation time (P = 0.55), postoperative complications (p = 0.11), and recurrence rate (P = 0.46), and the only difference is postoperative pain. DG-HAL causes less postoperative pain (P < 0.00001) [34]. A 705-patient multicenter study in Brazil found that a one-year follow-up after DG-HAL-RAR was significantly better in grades II and III compared to grade IV. Recurrence of prolapse, recurrence of bleeding, and thrombosis of grade II-III versus grade IV were 2.36% vs 26.54%, 1.01% vs 7.96%, and 1.35% vs 10.61%, respectively [35].

It should be noted that several conditions can contribute to increased pain after DG-HAL-RAR, namely the additional excision of thrombus of internal and external hemorrhoids, the presence of anal fissures, or laceration of the anal canal of the skin. This encourages caution during probe insertion. Additional local anesthetic infiltration will help to reduce postoperative pain [36]. In the case of large grade III and IV internal hemorrhoids, additional minimucosal excision is advised if any nodule remains after DG-HAL-RAR [37].

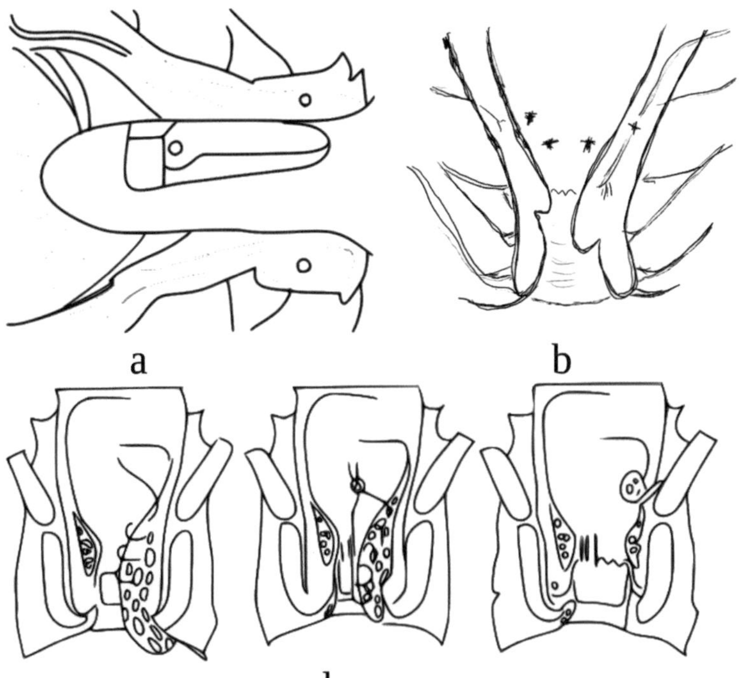

Figure 10.
DG-HAL-RAR a. Position of the probe to detect a branch of the superior rectal artery b. The number of arterial sutures varies from 5 to 8 and is not at the same level. c-d. Continues suturing for rectoanal repair. e. After the suture has been knotted, the final position. (Illustrated) by Kanaya).

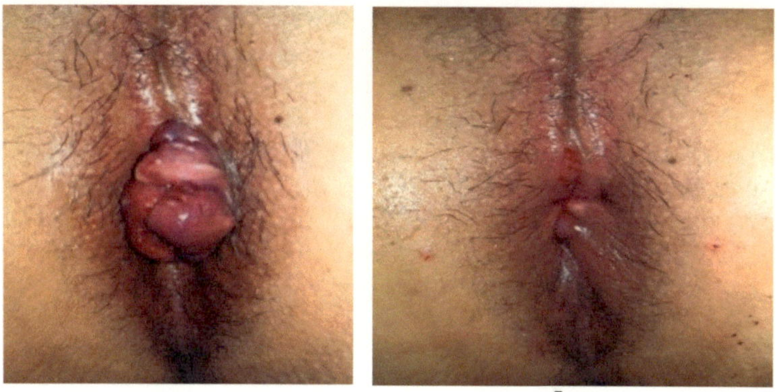

a b

Figure 11.
a. Prior to surgery, Grade III Internal Hemorrhoid, and b. After DG-HAL-RAR. (personal collection).

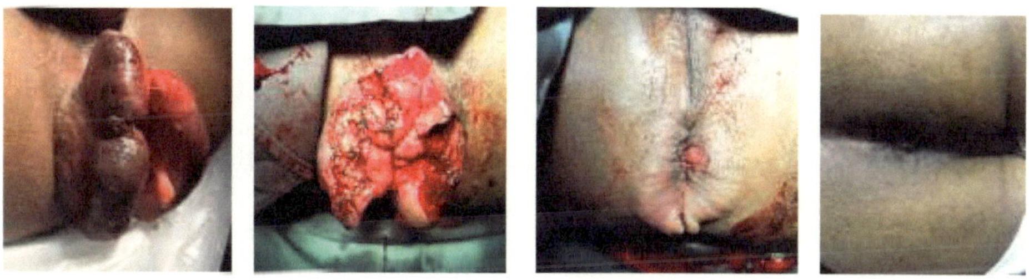

a b c d

Figure 12.
a. large circular Grade IV internal hemorrhoid, b. normal mucosal bridges are still visible after removal of three main piles (Milligan-Morgan Procedure). c. After DG-HAL-RAR of prominent visible mucosal bridges. d. 17 months postoperatively. (Personal collection).

In developing countries, cases of large circular Grade IV internal hemorrhoids occur very often (**Figure 12a**). Since the Whitehead procedure has already been abandoned due to its complications, the Morgan Milligan procedure is the only choice. However, after removing 3 main piles, the normal mucosal bridges are still prominent (**Figure 12b**). The addition of DG-HAL-RAR to prominent mucosal bridges gives a good result (**Figure 12c**). Followed up for 17 months, with a good appearance and no complaints (**Figure 12d**) [38].

6.15 Post-surgical care

For patients with instrumentation or surgery that only repositions the anal cushion, no special treatment is needed. Consuming high fiber and drinking lots of water will facilitate defecation, which is the standard for managing hemorrhoids, either conservatively or operatively, and also must be carried out postoperatively. The administration of analgesia is more tailored to the patient's needs because excision hemorrhoidectomy causes greater pain, so the need for analgesics is extra [2, 3]. Flavonoids, in this case, MPFF given post-surgery, have been proven by a meta-analysis of RCTs to reduce the risk of bleeding and post-surgical pain [14].

For excision hemorrhoidectomy, because the wound in the anal area, it requires special care. The anal area is a dirty area due to contamination with feces. Because of the pain, the patient will prefer not to wipe cleanly after defecation. Soaking in warm water with disinfectant will greatly help to clean the wound from contaminants, thereby helping reduce infection and speed healing. Soaking in warm water is also beneficial for reducing pain [8].

Changes in diet, method of defecation, and control of identified risk factors for the patients (chronic cough, shortness of breath, constipation, urinary difficulties, weight lifting, etc.) are important factors in preventing recurrence [8].

7. Summary

Hemorrhoids are frequently encountered in clinical practice, and physicians must be well-versed in the pathogenesis, risk factors, correct diagnosis, and correct management for patients to receive the best care and recover. The anal cushion sliding theory is now well accepted in the pathogenesis of hemorrhoids and is mostly related to constipation. Therefore, in the management of hemorrhoids, prevention or treatment of constipation has an important place. The first choice for preventing or treating constipation is to eat a high-fiber diet and drink plenty of water. Flavanoids, as oral medication, can be added since they have already been demonstrated to reduce hemorrhoid signs and symptoms. In the case of grades I, II, or small grades III, which fail in medicamentous treatment, instrumentation can be offered, and rubber band ligation is the best choice due to its effectiveness and low price. Surgery is the treatment of choice in emergency cases (thrombosis, strangulation, or bleeding that fails with other treatments) and in cases of grade III and IV that fail nonsurgical management. The gold standard of hemorrhoid surgery is excisional surgery, namely Morgan Milligan and Ferguson. Ferguson is slightly superior to Morgan Milligan regarding postoperative pain, bleeding, and speed of healing. Since excisional surgery is painful, nowadays it offers anal cushion preserving surgery. They are stapler hemorrhoidopexy (SH), hemorrhoidal artery ligation, and rectoanal repair under the guidance of Doppler (DG HAL-RAR). Both methods were comparable regarding the length of operative time, bleeding complications, and recurrence. But only regarding postoperative pain, DG HAL-RAR was superior to SH. DG HAL-RAR and SH also had less postoperative pain but higher recurrence compared to excisional surgery. Based on its advantages and disadvantages, let the patient choose the method of surgery.

Author details

Sigit Adi Prasetyo, Parish Budiono and Ignatius Riwanto*
Faculty of Medicine, Division of Digestive Surgery, Department of Surgery, Diponegoro University, Dr Kariadi General Hospital, Semarang, Indonesia

*Address all correspondence to: iriwanto@gmail.com

References

[1] Beck, DE, Steele, SR, & Wexner, SD. Fundamentals of Anorectal Surgery. 3rd ed. Philadelphia: Springer; 2019

[2] Lohsiriwat V. Hemorrhoids: From basic pathophysiology to clinical management World. Journal of Gastroenterology. 2012;**18**:2009-2017

[3] Ganz RA. The evaluation and treatment of hemorrhoids: A guide for the gastroenterologist. Clinical Gastroenterology and Hepatology. 2013;**11**:593-603

[4] Margetis N. Pathophysiology of internal hemorrhoids. Annals of Gastroenterology. 2019;**32**:264-272

[5] Aigner F, Gruber H, Conrad F, Eder J, Wedel T, Zelger B, et al. Revised morphology and hemodynamics of the anorectal vascular plexus: Impact on the course of hemorrhoidal disease. International Journal of Colorectal Disease. 2009;**24**(1):105-113

[6] Aigner F, Bodner G, Gruber H, Conrad F, Fritsch H, Margreiter R, et al. The vascular nature of hemorrhoids. Journal of Gastrointestinal Surgery. 2006;**10**(7):1044-1050

[7] Loder PB, Kamm MA, Nicholls RJ, Phillips KS. Haemorrhoids: Pathology, pathophysiology and aetiology. Brithish Journal of Surgery. 1994;**81**:946-954

[8] Davis BR, Lee-Kong SA, Migaly J, Feingold DL, Steele SR. The American Society of colon and rectal surgeons clinical practice guidelines for the management of hemorrhoids. Diseases of the Colon and Rectum. 2018;**61**:284-292

[9] Ratto C, Parello A, Donisi L. In: Litta F, editor. Colon, Rectum and Anus: Anatomic, Physiologic and Diagnostic Bases for Disease Management. Switzerland: Springer; 2017

[10] Malaguarnera G, Madeddu R, Catania VE, Bertino G, Morelli L, Perrotta RE, et al. Anorectal mucosal melanoma. Oncotarget. 2018;**9**(9): 8785-8800

[11] Alonso-Coello P, Mills E, Heels-Ansdell L-Y, Zhou Q, Johanson JF, et al. Fiber for the treatment of hemorrhoids complications: A systematic review and meta-analysis. The American Journal of Gastroenterology. 2006;**101**(1):181-188

[12] Lam TCF, Islam N, Lubowski DZ, King DW. Does squatting reduce pelvic floor descent during defecation? The Australian and New Zealand Journal of Surgery. 1993;**63**:172-174

[13] Periera N, Liolitsa D, Iype S, Croxford A, Yassin M, Lang P, et al. Phlebotonics for haemorrhoids (Review). The Cochrane Library. 2012;(8):1-59

[14] Sheikh P, Lohsiriwat V, Shelygin Y. Micronized purified flavonoid fraction in hemorrhoid disease: A systematic review and meta-analysis. Advances in Therapy. 2020;**37**:2792-2812

[15] Puspitasari. Pengaruh pemberian ekstrak daun wungu (Graptophyllum pictum GRIFT) dan Pegagan (Centella asiatica L) pada penderita hemoroid di desa Payaman Solokuro Lamongan. Airlangga University. 2016. Downloaded from: http://repository.unair.ac.id/30804/

[16] Prasetyo SA, Riwanto I, Dharmana E, Susilaningsih N, Prajoko YW, Nugroho EA. *Gratophyllum pictum* (L.) griff extract as anti-inflammatory on wistar rat with experimental hemorrhoids. study

on serum IL-6, COX-2, TNF-alpha and total leucocytes in anal tissue. International Surgery. 2020. DOI: 10.9738/INTSURG-D-18-00039.1

[17] Prasetyo SA, Wisnu Y, Nugroho EA, Dharmana E, Susilaningsih N, Riwanto I. Role of micronize purified flavonoid fraction and ethanol *Graptophyllum pictum* extract on experimental anal ulcer healing. Study on Wistar rat. Journal of Coloproctology. 2020;**4**:105-111

[18] Budiono BP, Prasetyo SA, Riwanto I, Susilaningsih N, Nugroho EA. *Graptophyllum pictum* extract in the treatment of experimental hemorrhoids: Effects on vascular leakage and matrix metalloproteinase-9 levels. Journal of Medical Sciences. 2021;**9**:1785-1789. DOI: 10.3889/oamjms.2021.7763

[19] Kaidar-Person O, Person B, Wexner SD. Hemorrhoidal disease: A comprehensive review. Journal of the American College of Surgeons. 2006;**204**(1): 102-117. DOI: 10.1016/j.jamcollsurg.2006.08.022. Epub 2006 Oct 25

[20] Johnson M. Trombosed Hemorrhoids 101: A Guide to Thrombosed Hemorrhoids Relief. 2017; Downlouded May 2021 from: https://senvie.com/blogs/senvie/thrombosed-hemorrhoids-guide-101

[21] Barwell J, Watkins RM, Lloyd-Davies E, Wilkins DC. Life-threatening retroperitoneal sepsis after hemorrhoid injection sclerotherapy: Report of a case. Diseases of the Colon and Rectum. 1999;**42**(3):421-423. DOI: 10.1007/BF02236364

[22] Maloku H, Gashi Z, Lazovic R, Islami H, Juniku-shkololli A. Laser hemorrhoidoplasty procedure vs open surgical hemorrhoidectomy: A trial comparing 2 treatments for hemorrhoids of third and fourth degree. Acta Informatica Medica. 2014 Dec;**22**(6):365-367

[23] Abiodun AA, Alatise OI, Okereke CE, Adesunkanmi ARK, Eletta EA, Gomna A. Comparative study of endoscopic band ligation versus injection sclerotherapy with 50% dextrose in water, in symptomatic internal haemorrhoids. The Nigerian Postgraduate Medical Journal. 2020;**27**:13-20

[24] van Tol RR, Bruijnen MPA, Melenhorst J, van Kuijk SMJ, Stassen LPS, Breukink SO. A national evaluation of the management practices of hemorrhoidal disease in the Netherlands. International Journal of Colorectal Disease. 2018;**33**:577-588

[25] Kanellos I, Goulimaris I, Christoforidis E, Kelpis T, Betsis DA. Comparison of the simultaneous application of sclerotherapy and rubber band ligation, with sclerotherapy and rubber band ligation applied separately, for the treatment of haemorrhoids: A prospective randomized trial. Colorectal Disease. 2003;**5**(2):133-138

[26] Bhatti MI, Sajid MS, Baig MK. Milligan–Morgan (Open) Versus Ferguson Haemorrhoidectomy (Closed): A Systematic Review and Meta-Analysis of Published Randomized Controlled Trials. World Journal of Surgery. 2016;**40**:1509-1519

[27] Devien CV. Death to Whitehead, hurray for Toupet or total circular Hemorrhoidectomy revisited. Its technique, their indications and their results. Annales de Chirurgie. 1994;**48**(6):565-571

[28] Li YD, Xu JH, Lin JJ, Zhu WF. Excisional hemorrhoidal surgery and its effect on anal continence. World Journal of Gastroenterology. 2012;**18**(30):4059-4063. DOI: 10.3748/wjg.v18.i30.4059

[29] Armstrong DN, Ambroze WL, Schertzer ME, Orangio GR. Harmonic scalpel vs. electrocautery prospective evaluation hemorrhoidectomy. Diseases of the Colon and Rectum. 2001;**4**(44):558-563

[30] Ratto C, Parello A, Donisi L, Litta F, Zaccone G, Doglietto GB. Assessment of haemorrhoidal artery network using colour duplex imaging and clinical implications. British Journal of Surgery. 2012;**99**:112-118

[31] Shao WJ, Li GCH, Zhang ZHK, Yang BL, Sun GD, Chen YQ. Systematic review and meta-analysis of randomized controlled trials comparing stapled haemorrhoidopexy with conventional haemorrhoidectomy. British Journal of Surgery. 2008;**95**:147-160

[32] Laughlan K, Jayne DG, Jackson D, Rupprecht F, Ribaric G. Stapled haemorrhoidopexy compared to Milligan–Morgan and Ferguson haemorrhoidectomy: A systematic review. International Journal of Colorectal Disease. 2009, 2009;**24**:335-344

[33] Ratto C. THD Doppler procedure for hemorrhoids: The surgical technique. Techniques in Coloproctology. 2014;**18**:291-298

[34] Sajid MS, Parampalli U, Whitehouse P, Sains P, McFall MR, Baig MKA. Systematic review comparing transanal haemorrhoidal de- arterialisation to stapled haemorrhoidopexy in the management of haemorrhoidal disease. Tech Coloproctology. 2012;**16**(1):1-8

[35] Sobrado CW, Klajner S, Hora JAB, Mello A, da Silva FML, Frugis MO, et al. Transanal haemorrhoidal dearterialization with mucopexy (Thd-M) for treatment of hemorrhoids: Is it applicable in all grades? Brazilian Multicenter Study. ABCD Arquivos Brasileros de Cirurgia Digestiva. 2020;**33**(2):e1504

[36] Prasetyo SA, Riwanto I. Factors affecting post-operative pain after doppler guided hemorrhoid artery ligation and recto-anal repair (DGHAL-RAR) of internal hemorrhoid. Media Medika Muda. 2016;**1**(3):145-150

[37] Theodoropoulos GE, Sevrisarianos N, Papaconstantinou J, Panoussopoulos SG, Dardamanis D, Stamapoulos P, et al. Doppler-guided haemorrhoidal artery ligation, rectoanal repair, sutured haemorrhoidopexy and minimal mucocutaneous excision for grades III-IV haemorrhoids: A multicenter prospective study of safety and efficacy. Colorectal Diseases. 2010;**12**(2):125-134

[38] Riwanto I, Prasetyo SA. Challenge in management prominent Grade IV hemorrhoid. In: Presented at 2nd MASTERCLASS in venous Disease for Asian Countries. The Athenee Hotel Bangkok, 27-28 January. 2018

Section 3

Pelvic Floor Disorder

Chapter 4

Efficiency of Treatment Targeted on Gut Microbiota in Inflammatory Bowel Diseases: Current Strategies and Perspectives

Daniela Cornelia Lazar, Elena-Alina Moacă, Mărioara Cornianu, Sorina Tăban, Alexandra Faur and Adrian Goldiș

Abstract

Inflammatory bowel diseases (IBDs) represent a category of diseases characterized by intestinal inflammation and include two main entities, ulcerative colitis and Crohn's disease, one of the representative clinical characteristics of which being chronic diarrhea. The etiology of these diseases is multifactorial, combining genetic, immunological, and also environmental factors, along with gut dysbiosis. In recent years, we encountered a higher incidence of IBD cases and of severe forms of disease. Therefore, there is an urgent need to develop new and efficient treatments, including strategies to improve the microbiome. In this chapter, we will discuss the current knowledge about the impact of different therapies influencing gut microbiota, such as prebiotics, probiotics, synbiotics, and other agents in IBD prevention, and also in the induction/maintenance of IBD remission. The manuscript will focus also on potential areas for research in the future using agents that modify intestinal microbiota and combined strategies.

Keywords: chronic diarrhea, inflammatory bowel diseases, microbiota, prebiotics, probiotics, synbiotics

1. Introduction

Inflammatory bowel diseases (IBDs) represent a category of diseases characterized by intestinal inflammation and include two main entities, ulcerative colitis and Crohn's disease, one of the representative clinical characteristics of which being chronic diarrhea. The etiology of these diseases is multifactorial, combining genetic, immunological, and also environmental factors, along with gut dysbiosis (**Figure 1**). In recent years, we encountered a higher incidence of IBD cases and of severe forms of disease. Therefore, there is an urgent need to develop new and efficient treatments, including strategies to improve the microbiome (**Figure 2**). In this chapter, we discuss

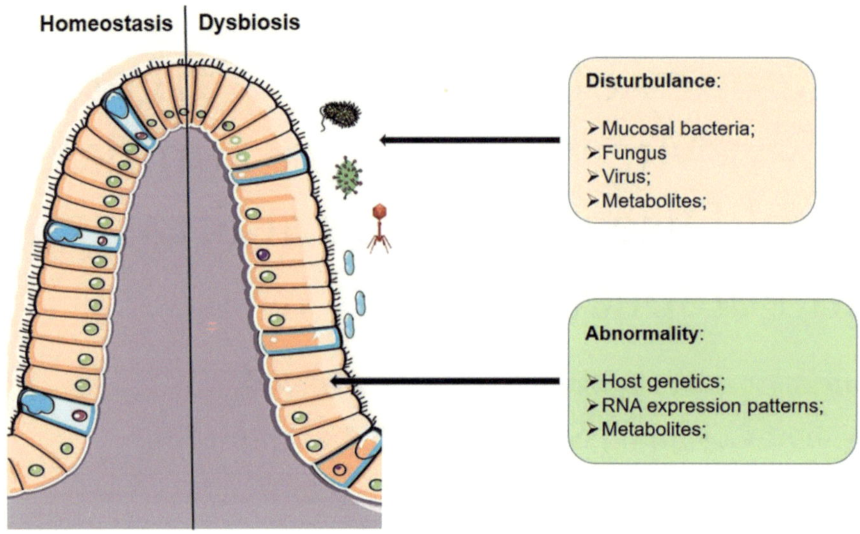

Figure 1.
The intestinal micro-environment dysbiosis in multi-dimension.

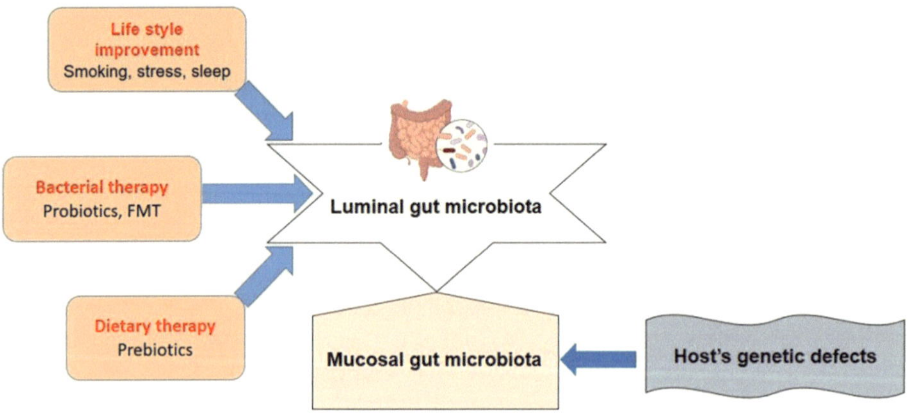

Figure 2.
Factors influencing microbiota.

the current knowledge about the impact of different therapies influencing gut microbiota, such as prebiotics, probiotics, synbiotics, and other agents in IBD prevention, and also in the induction/maintenance of IBD remission. The manuscript focuses also on potential areas for research in the future using agents that modify intestinal microbiota and combined strategies.

2. Gut microbiota modulation therapies

These therapies include different types of medical approaches; the chapter includes the most recent and relevant clinical data regarding the main strategies of treatment.

2.1 Nutritional therapies

2.1.1 Exclusive enteral nutrition (EEN)

This nutritional therapy has been recommended as first-line, steroid-sparing treatment for pediatric CD since the 1990s and provides the entire calorie and nutrient requirements using liquid formulations delivered either orally or through nasogastric tube or gastrostomy, for a period of 6–8 weeks. It is associated with remission rates of 60–80%, and the efficacy is not correlated with the formula types or the route of administration [1–6]. Most studies investigating the mechanism of action of EEN focused on the changes in gut flora and microbial metabolites as a potential mechanism, showing conflicting data. The first study on microbiota changes related to EEN used 16S ribosomal DNA polymerase chain reaction and temperature gradient gel electrophoresis and discovered important modification of the band profile associated with different bacterial species [7]. Later studies showed that although children treated with EEN had higher rates of mucosal healing, they still have a lower proportion of butyrate-producing bacteria in comparison with steroid-treated patients. A recent research revealed differences in the fecal metabolome of responders vs. non-responders to EEN [8, 9]. There are few data on the impact of EEN on the microbiota of adult CD patients; one study that investigated microbiota changes in adult CD patients treated with EEN for 2 weeks prior to intestinal resection for strictures found a significant decrease in alpha diversity and in the Enterobacteriaceae family, but which did not modify the postoperative recurrence [10].

2.2 Prebiotics and dietary fiber

Prebiotics are defined by the International Scientific Association for Probiotics and Prebiotics (ISAPP) as a “substrate that is selectively utilized by host microorganisms conferring a health benefit” [11, 12].

The most commonly used fibers in patients with digestive diseases are non-digestible soluble fibers that are fermented by the bacteria from the colon, leading to an increase in the concentration of some healthful bacterial metabolites such as short-chain fatty acids (SCFA). Soluble fiber, such as inulin, fructooligo- (FOS) and galactooligo-saccharides (GOS), lactulose and derivatives of galactose and β-glucans, proved to be efficient for the gut health, by both modulating gut microbiota and by exerting anti-inflammatory properties. These fibers can be naturally found in a huge number of products of plant origin and also added in different food products for nutritional and health purposes [6]. They increase the volume of the intestinal contents (by binding to water) and maintain the correct pH. Prebiotics increase the number of beneficial bacteria from the gut microbiome (i.e., the Lactobacillus, Bifidobacterium, and Bacteriodes families) and inhibit the pathogens [13, 14]. Also, they have a beneficial influence on the metabolism of lipids (lowers serum cholesterol level), glucose, and proteins, and increase the absorption of calcium, iron, and magnesium [11].

In order to be categorized as a prebiotic, a product must meet several conditions [12]:

- It should stimulate the proliferation and activity of some beneficial strains of gut bacteria

- It should create a favorable medium to some beneficial bacteria in the colon

- It should decrease the pH in the intestinal lumen
- It should be resistant to the action of digestive enzymes and process of hydrolysis
- It should not be absorbable in the upper digestive tract
- It should not be destroyed during the food processing process

2.2.1 Clinical studies on prebiotics in IBD

Research data demonstrate that prebiotics determine the change of gut microbiota spectrum and bacteria metabolites, but there are still few data published regarding prebiotics in IBD.

Benjamin et al. [15] performed a randomized, double-blind, placebo-controlled study, assessing the effect of FOS administration on active CD. The study was performed on 54 patients with CD and 49 controls; patients with active CD were randomized to receive FOS or placebo for a period of 4 weeks. Data showed a clinical worsening of the CD patients receiving prebiotics.

The results of another study showed that oral lactulose had no beneficial effect in active IBD (clinical, endoscopic, or histopathological activity), but it improves significantly the QoL in UC patients [16]. The multicenter clinical trial of Kanauchi et al. using germinated barley foodstuff (GBF) treatment in patients with mild-to-moderate active UC for 24 weeks showed significant improvement of clinical activity [17]. A research assessing the administration of inulin enriched with FOS in the same type of patients for 2 weeks demonstrated a significant reduction in the value of stool calprotectin [18].

Another study assessed the effect of GFB treatment for 12 months in inactive UC patients, revealing a lower rate of relapse [19]. A randomized, placebo-controlled study investigated the efficiency of ispaghula husk supplementation for 4 months in patients presenting inactive UC. They found a significantly higher rate of clinical improvement in the intervention group vs. placebo (69% vs. 24%) [20]. The study of Fernandez-Benarez investigated the effect of Plantago ovata seeds on three different groups of inactive UC (105 patients)—treated with mesalamine alone, Plantago ovata seeds with mesalamine, and Plantago ovata seeds alone for a period of 12 months, finding similar remission rates for all groups, but significant increase in stool butyrate levels in the groups treated with Plantago ovate [21].

To date, results of prebiotic research in patients with IBD are conflicting. Although the administration of prebiotic agents may be associated with some adverse digestive side effects in active IBD, their administration in early childhood for a proper development of gut microbiome and later prevention of IBD onset should be taken into consideration.

2.3 Probiotics

The human intestine is colonized by 10–100 trillion commensal bacteria that are involved in the digestion process, modulation of immune response, and other functions. Nowadays, due to excessive use of antibiotics, stress conditions, and hygiene, we encounter gut dysbiosis. Lactic-acid-producing bacteria (LAB) include the biggest part of the microbiome, which produce lactic acid as a result to the anaerobic digestion of saccharides. Lactobacillus spp. are the most important group of bacteria found in fermented food (e.g., pickles, soured milk, kefir) and are considered to be beneficial for humans [22, 23].

Probiotics are live organisms that are beneficial for the gut by modulating the immune response—increase the IgA production and enhance the host immune system`s defenses—and are able to compete with pathogens [24, 25]. Their favorable actions on human gut are the following [26–29]:

- The production of components with antibacterial activity (e.g., lactic acid, bacteriocins, hydroperoxides)
- Competitively block the binding sites on the epithelial cells and upregulate tight junction molecules of the mucosal barrier
- The degradation of the receptors for toxins
- Change of intestinal pH
- Competition for essential nutrients

The beneficial effect of probiotics was known through antibiotic-based therapy [30, 31] to decrease blood cholesterol level [32], the treatment of local infections [33], and others. In case of IBD patients, there is an abnormal activation of the immune system due to chronic intestinal inflammation. Prebiotics modulate the immune system in the mucosa layer of the intestine, by stimulating the production of antibodies, promoting phagocytosis and NK activity, determining T cell apoptosis, enhancing anti-inflammatory cytokines while reducing the pro-inflammatory ones.

2.3.1 Clinical studies and meta-analysis with probiotics in IBD

The randomized double-blind study by Tamaki et al. [24] performed in patients with mild/moderate UC demonstrated a reduction in clinical activity assessed by Ulcerative Colitis Activity Score (UCDAI), though not reaching statistical significance, in 28 patients treated with Bifidobacterium longum 536 vs. 28 patients in the placebo group, after 8 weeks of follow-up. They observed a statistically significant improvement in rectal bleeding and endoscopic activity assessed by Mayo scale.

A single-center, randomized, double-blind and placebo-controlled study [34] in patients with UC in clinical remission compared a group of patients treated with Bio-Three (Streptococcus faecalis T-110, Clostridium butyricum TO-A, and Bacillus mesentericus TO-A), with a placebo group for a period of 1 year, demonstrated lower relapsing rate in the study group, but statistically significance was reached only at 3 months of study. Yilmaz et al. [35] performed a prospective open-label randomized control, single-center study that assessed the administration of fermented milk (400 ml of kefir daily) for 4 weeks. Their results showed a statistically significant reduction of the inflammatory syndrome, improvement of hemoglobin level, and results of good feeling score, in both CD and UC patients from the study group in comparison with controls. The randomized, placebo-controlled trial of Shadnoush et al. [36] on IBD patients remarked significantly higher amounts of Lactobacillus, Bifidobacterium, and Bacteroides in patients treated with yogurt vs. control group after 8 weeks.

A study compared effect of the treatment with mesalazine and a probiotic blend (Lactobacillus salivarius, Lactobacillus acidophilus, and Bifidobacterium bifidus BGN4) vs. mesalazine alone for 24 month in patients with moderate-to-severe UC demonstrated a statistically significant improvement in endoscopic activity and clinical symptoms in the first group vs. the group with aminosalicylates treatment, suggesting that the combined treatment could be a feasible alternative to steroid treatment [37]. Another study [38] compared a group treated with mesalazine and Bifico (containing Enterococcus faecalis, Bifidobacterium longum, and Lactobacillus acidophilus) vs. a group treated with mesalazine alone. After 40 days of treatment, a significant reduction in Enterobacteria, Enterococci, Saccharomyces, and Bacteroides and increases in Bifidobacteria and Lactobacilli, and also lower levels of CRP, fecal lactoferrin, alpha-1-antitrypsin and beta-2-microglobulin, IL-6, and higher level of IL-4 in the study group were noticed. The study of Su et al. [39] randomized patients with CD to two study groups, one treated with probiotics (Bifidobacterium and Lactobacillus) combined with sulfasalazine and prednisone and the other one treated with sulfasalazine alone, which were further compared with a healthy control group. Authors noticed a significant reduction in the pro-inflammatory cytokines, better therapeutic efficiency, and lower infection rate in the study group.

Bjarnason et al. [40] randomized 81 patients with UC and 61 with CD into two groups, one using multistrain probiotic agent named Symprove that contains Lactobacillus rhamnosus NCIMB 30174, Lactobacillus plantarum NCIMB 30173, Lactobacillus acidophilus NCIMB 30175, and Enterococcus faecium NCIMB 30176 with a second group of placebo. They noticed a statistically significant improvement in the level of fecal calprotectin in patients with UC treated with multistrain probiotic agent, without significant differences in other parameters. The multi-center, randomized, placebo-controlled study of Fedorak et al. [41] on 120 patients with CD who underwent ileocolonic surgical resection compared the study group treated with VLS#3 (an agent that contains viable bacteria, including four strains of Lactobacillus combined with three strains of Bifidobacterium and one strain of Streptococcus salivarius subspecies thermophilus) vs. a placebo group. After 1 year of follow-up, there were found lower rates of severe endoscopic recurrence and significant reductions in pro-inflammatory cytokine levels in the study group treated with VLS#3 vs. control group.

One study evaluated the effect of administration of the Bifidobacterium breve strain Yakult (BFM) found in fermented milk in patients with UC vs. placebo regarding the relapse-free survival and incidence of relapse, but they found no significant differences [42].

Asto et al. [43] performed a meta-analysis in which they evaluated 18 placebo-controlled studies (1997–2018), including 1491 patients with UC who were treated with prebiotics, probiotics, or synbiotics vs. placebo groups; although any significant effect in maintaining remission was not demonstrated, it could be concluded that probiotics are beneficial in achieving remission in the active phase of UC. The results of the meta-analysis of Zhang et al. [44] comprising 38 studies demonstrated that probiotics, prebiotics, and synbiotics are efficient in achieving and maintaining remission, and their use determined a reduction in UC disease activity index. Probiotics lead to an increase in the number of intestinal Bifidobacteria, and synbiotics were more efficient in comparison with probiotics and prebiotics.

The meta-analysis of Jia et al. [45] included 10 studies (1999–2013), most of them focusing on *E. coli* Nissle and VSL#3. The results demonstrated significant differences between *E. coli* Nissle vs. mesalazine in the remission rate, risk of recurrence, and occurrence of complications; also, statistically significant higher rates of remission and lower risk of recurrence were obtained with VLS#3 vs. control groups. Puvvada et al. [46] analyzed three RCTs, which examined the effect of probiotics on the QoL of patients with IBD (two of them with positive results). The authors concluded that probiotics have beneficial effects of the QoL of IBD patients.

2.3.2 Side effects of probiotics

The meta-analysis of Dore et al. [47] on the incidence of side effects related to the use of probiotics in IBD patients that included nine trials (826 patients) demonstrated a higher percentage of side effects in the group of patients treated with probiotics; this effect was remarked only in patients with UC, but not with CD. These studies referred to more digestive side effects, abdominal pain occurring significantly more often in patients using probiotics. Later (2020), the same group performed a retrospective cohort study on IBD patients, 100 taking probiotics (VSL#3, Lactobacillus reuteri, and a mixture of S. thermophiles and L. acidophilus, B. breve and B. animalis ssp. Lactis) and 100 controls, showing that the incidence of adverse effects (need for systemic steroids, hospitalization, and surgery) was lower in patients taking probiotics (more than 75% of the duration of IBD) and especially in UC patients [48].

Probiotics are commonly considered as safe agents, reducing the adverse effects of the IBD, but we have to keep in mind that exceptionally, in immunosuppressed patients, bacterial translocation and sepsis may develop.

2.3.3 Probiotic engineering in the treatment of IBD

The use of probiotics helps the transition from a pro-inflammatory to an anti-inflammatory state at the gut level. Nowadays, the strains currently available as probiotics are represented by the Bifidobacterium species, Enterococcus faecium, Lactobacillus strains, Saccharomyces boulardii, Bacillus species, and Pediococcus, which have been demonstrated to be associated with the beneficial health effects [27, 49, 50]. Probiotic engineering determines the formation of bacterial strains with more powerful properties to target the enteric pathogens and to specifically intervene in IBD. These types of probiotics have the capacity to synthesize in situ a one or multitude of desired therapeutic biomolecules able to act on gut inflammation and avoid the side effects and complications associated with current treatment. This strategy uses bacteria or yeasts genetically engineered with the genes for some therapeutic agents that are acting as anti-inflammatory agents [22, 51].

One of the strategies used in probiotic engineering used a xylan-inducible system in Bacteriodes ovatus, which was able to induce some important biomolecules for the maintaining of gut integrity [52].

Many cytokines have been involved in IBD. Lactococcus lactis has been engineered to produce anti-inflammatory cytokine IL-10 [53]. IL-10 treatment proved to be promising in animal models of IBD and also in clinical trials using IBD patients [49]. Results of two trials performed by IBD Cooperative Study Group demonstrated an improvement of the disease in 23.5% of patients receiving IL-10 vs. placebo [54–58]. IL-27 is known to play a crucial role in infectious diseases, autoimmunity, and cancer in many organs and systems, including the digestive tract. In an animal model, treatment with IL-27 was able to diminish experimental colitis. Moreover, in colitis mouse models, engineered IL-27-producing L. lactis demonstrated to be more efficient than both the IL-10-producing L. lactis and systemic administration of IL-27 [59–61].

Interleukin 35 (IL-35) is an anti-inflammatory cytokine from the IL-12 family and plays an important role in immune suppression. IL-35 plays a pivotal role in the development and the function of both regulatory B (Bregs) and T cells (Tregs). IL-35 functions as a new anti-inflammatory factor for IBD and other immune diseases. Therapeutic potential of recombinant IL-35 protein was assessed in DSS-induced colitis mouse model. Recombinant IL-35 protein could slow down the pathologic process in mouse model. Trefoil factors (TFF) and anti TNF-α nanobodies (single domain antibody fragments) represent other therapeutic agents that have been constitutively expressed in L. lactis and tested in DSS-induced colitis in mice [49]. The former have protective and reparative properties on the intestinal epithelium. The peptides produced *in situ* by L. lactis were considerably more effective at healing colitis than the oral or rectal administration of the purified TFF [49].

One recent study engineered E. coli Nissle 1917 to produce an extracellular matrix including all three trefoil factors in order control inflammation. Tumor necrosis factor (TNF) is a pro-inflammatory cytokine secreted in IBD, and antibodies for this cytokine are used nowadays as a treatment for IBD, but associated with some side effects and disadvantages. Oral administration of nanobody-secreting L. lactis leads in local delivery of anti-mTNF nanobodies in the gut and was associated with a significant reduction of inflammation in a mouse model of DSS-induced colitis. This way of administration has been proved to prevent the systemic side effects of anti-TNF through localized delivery [62].

2.3.4 Probiotic engineering in vaccinations

Traditional oral vaccinations may fail to resist in the harsh gastric environment and, sometimes, they are unable to act on the most important immune structures that induce immunity. Furthermore, there is the possibility of reversion to a virulent state of the attenuated microbes [63]. On the other hand, engineered probiotics have the following advantages:

- are able to deliver medication/vaccinations where these types of vaccinations are effective in inducing intestinal immunity
- are more easier to store and are much cheaper than the conventional biologics [64]
- have increased survival potential under unfavorable environmental conditions
- can be manipulated to determine a tolerogenic immune response
- can be specifically targeted to some immune structures such as Peyer's patches [65].

But we have to take into considerations several disadvantages related to safety concerns. Bioengineered probiotics represent microbes and are genetically modified organisms (GMO) [66]; therefore, they pose some challenge for the approval of administration. Moreover, patients may be skeptic about their safety and their effects on the environment. To prevent bacterial gene transfer and survival in the natural medium, specific guidelines and containment strategies as well as specific engineering methods can be developed.

2.4 Synbiotics

Synbiotics represents a combination of prebiotics and probiotics with synergistic beneficial effect, but for now there are still few literature data on their effect on IBD patients; more often, they contain Lactobacillus GG and/or Bifidobacteria combined with FOS and/or inulin [67, 68]. In the double-blind trial of Steed et al. [69], patients with active CD were randomized to receive 6 g per day of either a synbiotic (a combination of inulin and FOS) vs. placebo for 6 months. The results demonstrated significant reduction in the clinical and histopathological activity of CD, an increased population of Bifidobacteria species in the study group, and a decrease in TNF alpha after 3 months (but not 6 months). Another randomized, double-blind and placebo-controlled study [70] evaluated the same symbiotic for a period of 1 month, revealing significant improvement in the endoscopic and histopathological activity in the rectal biopsies and reduction in serum CRP, TNF-α, and IL-1 α and mucosal human beta defensins 2, 3, 4.

The randomized, double-blind and placebo-controlled trial of Chermesh et al. [71] investigated Synbiotic 2000 including four probiotics and four prebiotics administrated for 24 months found no significant differences between the study group and placebo regarding clinical picture, laboratory data, and endoscopic activity. Fujimori et al. [72] included 120 patients with UC (active and inactive) that were randomized into three groups, first treated with probiotic (Bifidobacterium longum), the second with prebiotic (Psyllium), and the third one with symbiotic (bifidobacterium longum plus psyllium) for 4 weeks, observing a significant improvement in the QoL and decrease in CRP level in the group treated with symbiotic vs. the other two groups. Another study investigated 41 patients with mild-to-moderate UC, randomized into two groups, one with standard treatment associated with symbiotic (Bifidobacterium breve strain Yakult plus GOS) vs. the second group treated only with standard treatment. After 1 year of treatment, authors noticed significant reduction in clinical and endoscopic activity in study group vs. control [73].

2.5 Paraprobiotics

Paraprobiotics are represented by dead probiotic bacteria cells and cell constituents. The idea of treating with inactivated bacterial strains or fragments or even bacterial metabolite products instead of probiotics is reasonable taking into consideration the risk of administrating probiotics in sepsis, immunosuppressed subjects, and premature babies [74, 75]. They are manufactured by cultivating selected strains of bacteria and their subsequent inactivation [76, 77].

The advantages of paraprobiotic administration are the following [78–80]:

- the absence of risk of bacterial translocation
- the absence of risk of transferring antibiotic resistance genes
- are easier to produce, transport, and store
- more precise therapeutic effects due to their administration in adequate amounts
- possibility to be used even in preterm neonates` treatment
- multidirectional way of action, the most important being immunomodulation

Several highly efficient bacterial strains for the health have been selected to be used as paraprobiotics: Bifidobacterium lactis Bb12, Bifidobacterium longum, Lactobacillus gasseri OLL2716, Lactobacillus brevis SBC8803, and Lactobacillus delbrueckii subsp. bulgaricus OLL1073R-1 and Saccharomyces cerevisiae. Moreover, proteins and peptides, polysaccharides (glucans), and fragments of genetic material in the form of AT DNA obtained from Lactobacillus spp. have similar effects [81].

At the moment, there are several *in vitro* studies demonstrating the beneficial immunomodulatory effect of paraprobiotics in IBD patients. Also, some of the paraprobiotic proteins can improve the regeneration of the intestinal mucosa, and yeast cell wall components may improve digestion.

In vitro studies demonstrated immunomodulatory, anti-inflammatory, antiproliferative, and antioxidant effects of paraproteins, which seem to be able to prevent and improve the clinical symptoms of IBD patients [82–84].

2.6 Postbiotics

The term postbiotics refers to metabolites and cell-free supernatants (CFS) and also soluble factors such as metabolic bioproducts secreted by live microbes [80]. Metabiotics refers to the structural constituents of probiotic bacteria and/or their metabolites and/or specific signaling molecules that can improve physiological functions of the body and regulatory or metabolic reactions related with gut microbiota [85, 86].

Postbiotics are found in fermented food (kefir, sauerkraut, yogurt, certain pickles, etc.) and inside the human body. They are mainly represented by organic acids (i.e., short-chain fatty acids (SCFA)), tryptophan (Trp), and bacteriocins and present direct benefits due to their action on the host cells and indirect benefits related to the stimulation of proliferation of beneficial gut bacterial strains and inhibition of harmful microbial strains. They may have different properties depending on their type; the most important benefit is related to their anti-inflammatory and antioxidant effects.

2.6.1 SCFAs

They are produced by the intestinal fermentation of dietary fiber, non-starch polysaccharides (NSP), and resistant starch, mainly in the proximal part of the large bowel, in relationship with the substrates and the microbiota. The most important SCFAs are represented by acetic acid (AA), propionic acid (PA), and butyric acid (BA), and a proper SCFA ratio helps the immune system. Also, they have the capacity to acidify the environment, which is considered by some researchers to be beneficial by improving the bioavailability of metals and by protecting against the pathogenic bacteria, but harmful by others due to the supposed damage of the intestinal mucosal barrier [87–90].

2.6.1.1 Butyric acid (BA)

BA represents one of the most potent SCFAs, acting both in intestinal and parenteral way [91].

The complex intestinal effects of BA are the following [92–95]:

- represents one of the primary energy sources for colonocytes
- has a protective intestinal effect by enhancing the expression of mucin genes and mucin production

- stimulates the proliferation of normal enterocytes and inhibits the proliferation of cancerous cells ("butyrate paradox") secondary to the inhibition of histone deacetylase (HDAC)

- decreases the expression of genes involved in the synthesis of the major pro-inflammatory cytokines by inhibiting the activity of the NF-κB complex in the immune cells

- presents an antioxidant effect by increasing the level of reduced glutathione

At the moment, there are inconclusive results of the clinical studies using either rectal infusions or oral formulas with BA in patients with IBD.

The parenteral effect of BA, produced also though the inhibition of HDAC, consists of [96–98]:

- stimulates hemoglobin synthesis and increases the number of reticulocytes, therefore leading to amelioration of anemia in IBD patients

- determines the secretion of anti-inflammatory cytokine IL-10 and aldehyde dehydrogenase by binding to a specific receptor expressed in adipocites and immune cells

- enhances the detoxification process and the removal of electrophilic compounds in association to the stimulation of Treg lymphocyte differentiation

2.6.1.2 Propionic acid (PA)

PA is found naturally in dairy products secondary to the natural fermentation by Propionibacterium and also may be added as food preservative. PA produced in the intestine by the fermentation process of different compounds determined by anaerobic flora comprises a much higher proportion compared with the amount delivered with food [99]. The effects of PA reside in [11, 100]:

- antibacterial and antifungal effects—it inhibits the genes of pathogenic bacteria and prevents gut colonization with pathogens from Sallmonela family

- inhibition of local inflammation by diminishing COX2 enzymes and formation of prostaglandins

- anti-inflammatory properties:

    - inhibits lymphocyte proliferation

    - activates the synthesis of anti-inflammatory resistin in adipose tissue

    - inhibits TNF-α release by neutrophils and endothelial cells

    - represents the most potent ligand of GPCR43, a receptor exposed to immunocites, proving a strong relationship with the immune system

2.6.1.3 Acetic acid (AA)

There are discordant results concerning AA, some research suggesting stimulation of the proliferation of neoplastic tissue, others inhibition of the neoplastic tissue during hypoxia, and even onset of metabolic syndrome and obesity [101, 102].

2.6.1.4 Adjuvant treatment with SCFA in IBD

Vernia et al. [103] used enemas twice daily for a period of 6 weeks vs. placebo group; they obtained statistically significant decreases in intestinal bleeding and urgency, as well as an improved patient self-evaluation score compared with placebo. The study of Lührs et al. [104] compared the efficiency of a butyrate enema versus a placebo, used twice daily for a period of 8 weeks. They showed that study patients presented a significant reduction in the number of macrophages with NF-kB expression and also a decreased number of neutrophils in crypt and epithelia and of lymphocytes and plasma cells of the lamina propria, proved in bioptic specimens, in correlation with the disease activity. Another study performed a randomized, prospective evaluation of corticosteroid enemas and mesalazine enemas vs. SCFA enemas in patients with distal UC (proctosigmoiditis), proving similar recovery rates between these three groups [105].

The study of Hamer et al. [93] using rectal enemas with sodium butyrate vs. saline for 20 days in patients presenting distal UC in clinical remission demonstrated minor effects induced by butyrate on colonic inflammation and oxidative stress. They proved the effect of BA on colonic glutathione levels. Another randomized trial [106] investigated sodium butyrate enemas for 2 weeks vs. placebo in patients with distal UC non-responsive to conventional treatment. The authors found a significant decrease in the number of stools, blood discharge, endoscopic score of severity, and histologic score of inflammation in patients treated with SCFA enemas. Scheppach et al. [107] compared enemas of combined SCFA, butyrate, or saline placebo in patients with active distal UC twice daily for 8 weeks showing a trend toward a beneficial effect of SCFA enemas. Some other studies were not able to prove the efficiency of treatment with SCFA enemas [108, 109]. They were able to show that only patients with colitis dating back less than 6 months responded significantly more to SCFA vs. placebo. In conclusion, the results of most studies using SFCA are inconsistent.

2.6.2 Tryptophan (Trp)

Tryptophan represents a fine regulator of inflammation involved in the adaptive immunity, mucosal barrier, and intestinal homeostasis. Gut microbiota metabolizes tryptophan, through this influencing serotonin and the immune system. Most products of the bacterial metabolism of tryptophan represent ligands for the aryl hydrocarbon receptor (AhR) that mediate the expression of genes responsible for the metabolism of xenobiotics (i.e., dioxins, drugs) metabolized by the cytochrome P450. Tryptophan metabolites such as AhR ligands are essential in the gut mucosal protection against inflammation and for maintaining intestinal homeostasis by helping mucosal barrier integrity and acting on many immune cell types. The metabolism of Trp generates some bioactive postbiotic derivatives, including indole acetate and propionate indole. Host enzymes involved in Trp metabolism (IDO1 enzyme) have a positive effect on clinical activity of IBD [110–114].

In patients with IBD, it was suggested that pro-inflammatory cytokines initiate the conversion of Trp to its metabolites. A very small amount of ingested Trp is conversed to serotonin, which acts not only on the CNS but also on the digestive tract, influencing gut vasodilation, motility, secretion, and absorption processes. Trp and its metabolites represent potential therapeutic targets in IBD. In this regard, trials using the administration of Lactobacillus, which produces AhR agonists, were able to demonstrate a decrease of colonic inflammation in animal models [115, 116].

2.7 Antibiotics

Antibiotics may have an insecure effect on the gut microbiota homeostasis, leading to an increase in Enterobacteriaceae and reduction in Clostridia, representing a possible pre-IBD state [117]. Moreover, IBD patients treated with antibiotics have an increased risk of developing an overgrowth of pathogenic microbes (e.g., Clostridioides difficile), fungi (e.g., candida), and bacteriophages [118]. Antibiotics have been widely used, in both pediatric and adult IBD especially in situations (pouchitis, perianal disease, abdominal abscesses), but even in luminal disease. Suggested potential mechanisms for the role of antibiotics in IBD patients include [119, 120]:

- direct influence on the gut microbiota, stimulating anti-inflammatory flora (e.g., Bacteroides and Firmicutes), while reducing bacteria that are associated with inflammation (Enterobacteriaceae—Escherichia coli, Fusobacterium)
- change metabolic enzymatic pathways determined by gut bacteria
- target pathobionts that are invading the mucosa in CD

In most of the cases, antibiotics are used empirically, without identification of a specific microbial target. A case series [121] with very early-onset IBD patients refractory to other conventional treatments, mean age of 1.6 years, demonstrated that oral administration of Vancomycin ± Gentamycin can induce sustained remission.

The Cochrane systematic review of Townsend et al. [122] assessed the efficacy and safety of antibiotic administration for induction/maintenance of remission in CD. There were 13 RCTs included, comprising 1303 patients. Comparisons included ciprofloxacin/rifaximin/metronidazole/clarithromycin/cotrimoxazole vs. placebo, ciprofloxacin plus metronidazole vs. methylprednisolone, ciprofloxacin, metronidazole and budesonide vs. placebo with budesonide, ciprofloxacin vs. mesalazine, ciprofloxacin plus adalimumab vs. placebo with adalimumab, ciprofloxacin plus infliximab vs. placebo with infliximab, clarithromycin and antimycobacterial vs. placebo, and metronidazole plus cotrimoxazole vs. placebo. All antibiotics were pooled as a class vs. placebo, and antibiotics plus anti-TNF vs. placebo with anti-TNF. There was an uncertain effect of individual antibiotics on CD patients due to imprecision. Considering antibiotics as a class, 55% of the patients treated with antibiotic failed to achieve remission at 6–10 weeks vs. 64% of placebo group; 41% of the patients with antibiotic failed to achieve a clinical response at 10–14 weeks vs. 49% of placebo group (RR 0.77). The effect of antibiotics on relapse and on serious AE was unclear. They do not seem to increase the risk of AEs. The most frequent adverse events included gastrointestinal distress, upper respiratory tract infection, abscess development, headache, change in taste, and paresthesia. When antibiotics were combined with anti-TNF, 21% of patients on associated therapy failed to achieve a clinical response/remission at week 12 vs. 36% of placebo patients (RR 0.57, low certainty evidence); 77% of the combined group had an AE compared with 83% with placebo (RR 0.93). In active CD, evidence suggests a modest benefit provided by antibiotics that may not be clinically significant. In this context, more research is needed to establish the efficacy and safety of antibiotic treatment for maintenance of remission in CD patients.

In the future, due the development of microbiome evaluation techniques, by assessing the specific gut microbiome from patient stool samples before treatment, we will be able to select the right IBD candidates for antimicrobial treatment [123] in order to target specific pathobionts or to favorable modulate microbiome/metabolome.

2.8 Fecal microbiota transplantation (FMT) for the treatment of IBD

The study of Zhang et al. [124] investigating the role of FMT in an UC mouse model induced by dextran sulfate sodium demonstrated that FMT intervention decreased disease activity index levels and the histopathological changes, reduced the expression of colonic cytokines and oxidative stress, restored the gut microbiota, and increased the concentrations of gut SCFAs.

The systematic review of Imdad et al. [125] included four studies (277 participants), which assessed the efficiency of FMT for the treatment of UC, most of the subjects presenting mild-moderate forms of disease; authors did not find any eligible trials for the treatment of CD. Three of the studies administered FMT *via* the rectal route and one study *via* the nasoduodenal route. Combined data suggest that FMT increases the percentage of clinical remission by twofold in patients with UC compared with control group, 37% (52/140) of FMT patients vs. 18% (24/137) of control subjects achieving remission (RR 2.03). One of the studies reported that none of the patients receiving FMT relapsed at 12 weeks vs. 20% of control (RR 0.28). It was inconclusive whether there is a difference in serious adverse event (SAE) rates between the FMT and control groups, including worsening of the disease needing intravenous steroids/surgery, infections (e.g., Clostridium difficille, cytomegalovirus), small bowel perforation, and pneumonia. Common adverse events included digestive symptoms, upper respiratory tract infection, fever, headache, and dizziness. At 8 weeks, 49% (68/140) of FMT patients vs. 28% (38/137) of controls achieved clinical response (RR 1.70). Also, 30% (35/117) of FMT vs. 10% (11/112) of control subjects (RR 2.96) achieved endoscopic remission.

The systematic review and meta-analysis of Fang et al. [126] investigated the efficacy and safety and protocol of FMT for IBD, including a total of 596 pediatric and adult patients, out of which 459 received FMT. Data showed that patients with moderate-severe attacks of disease could develop significantly higher remission rates with FMT vs. patients with mild-moderate attacks. Also, in case of UC patients, FMT determined significantly higher clinical remission rates vs. placebo (28% vs. 9%, P=0.0003). The authors conclude that FMT represents an efficient and safe therapy for IBD patients (both pediatric and adult). In this meta-analysis, the type of donor stool (fresh/frozen), route of delivery, and antibiotic pretreatment proved to have no impact in patients with IBD. Due to these results, they considered FMT as a potential rescue therapy, possibly even an initial therapy for IBD.

Sokol et al. [127] performed a randomized, single-blind and sham-controlled pilot study of FMT in adults with colonic/ileocolonic CD who were enrolled while receiving oral corticosteroid in active disease. After achieving clinical remission, patients were randomized to receive either FMT or sham transplantation, while receiving a second colonoscopy at week 6. The primary endpoint consisted of the implantation of the donor microbiota at week 6 (Sorensen index > 0.6). In this study, eight patients received FMT and nine patients sham transplantation. Data revealed that none of the patients included reached the primary endpoint. Because a low similarity index between donor and recipient gut microbiota in several patients was detected, authors assume that a single FMT might not be sufficient to induce significant changes. However, FMT demonstrated to be more efficient over sham transplantation in decreasing Crohn's Disease Endoscopic Index of Severity (CDEIS) and CRP level, and a higher colonization by donor microbiota leads to the maintenance of remission. These results must be confirmed in larger studies.

At this time, we can conclude that, although there were some clinical benefits seen in UC patients treated with FMT, there is still some uncertainty regarding the rate of serious adverse events related to FMT treatment in IBD patients. Moreover, further studies are needed to evaluate the efficacy of FMT treatment for induction of remission in CD patients (**Figure 3**). Future research should define the optimal parameters of FMT (delivery route, frequency, volume, type of preparation, type of donor, and also the type of IBD and severity of the attack). Also, more data regarding long-term maintenance of remission with FMT treatment in IBD patients are needed, along with validation regarding long-term safety of FMT.

2.9 Phage therapy

Research studies assessed the association of the enteric virome and IBD, showing alterations of the virome patients with IBD. One study showed an increased

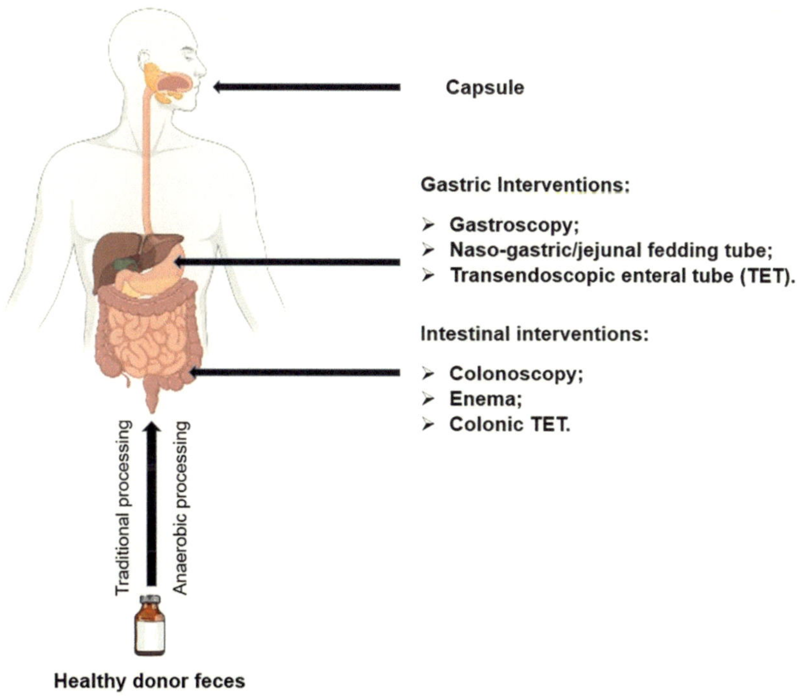

Figure 3.
Fecal microbiota transplantation regimen.

number of phages infecting some bacteria such as Clostridiales, Alteromonadales, and Clostridium acetobutylicum, along with a higher number of viruses from the Retroviridae family in IBD patients [128, 129]. A follow-up study identified a significantly higher diversity from phages associated with a reduction in bacterial diversity in subjects with IBD vs. controls. In a pediatric population with IBD, Caudovirales were more significantly represented [130]. Higher abundance and reduced diversity of phages and a decreased number of phage-related functions in patients with UC [131] were discovered; these aspects suggest the possibility of new treatments targeting the virome in this IBD subtype.

"Phage therapy" signifies the modulation of phageome, and by this, the bacteriome of an individual suffering from a disease considered to stem from bacterial origin (**Figure 4**). It includes several steps [132]:

- changing the genetic information of an existing phage for successful adsorption to a specific bacterial strain
- preparation of one/more phage strains
- development of a dosing schedule
- administration of the preparation to the patient

In this regard, phages engineered to be usable for treatment should not be recognized by the immune system of the host. Several studies revealed the ability of phages to stimulate the production of antibodies, findings that could assign phages negative effects on the gut environment. However, there are data showing that phages may also have anti-inflammatory effects. For example, the modulation of NF-κB activity by Staphylococcus aureus phage was discovered [133]. It is considered that the systemic presence of phages could play a crucial role in diminishing the immune response and the development of some auto inflammatory/inflammatory diseases including IBD.

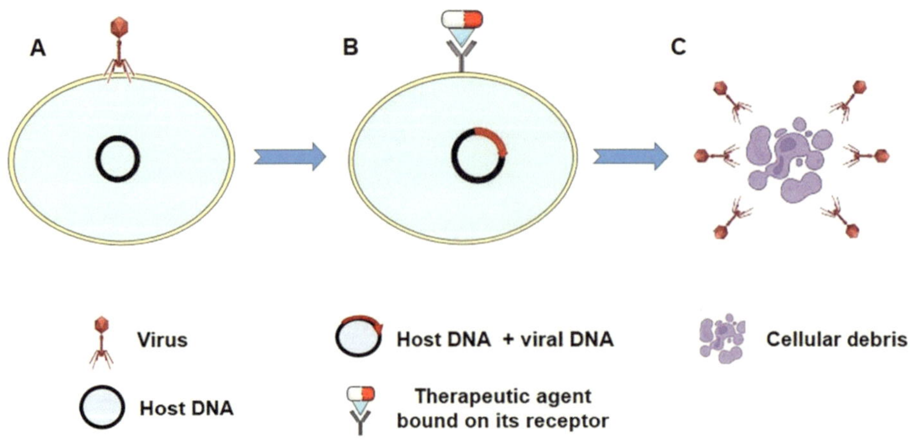

Figure 4.
Phage therapy modulation. A—the phage attachments to the host; the incorporation of the genetic information into the DNA of the host; B—the administration of the therapeutic agent; C—the degradation of the bacterium.

Górski et al. found that the phages can traverse the mucosa and enter the systemic circulation, a phenomenon discovered even in healthy subject and associated with immunomodulation [134]. Inflammation increases the intestinal permeability, and a higher number of phages enter in the circulation.

In an IBD patient, it was considered important to be able to introduce a "phage cocktail" into the colon that is not able to incorporate its genetic information into bacteria. Therefore, phages may be engineered to lack the enzyme determining the genome integration [135]. On the other hand, it may be more useful to control the switch between lytic/lysogenic life cycles, as it might be more beneficial if the phage stayed incorporated in the gut bacterial genome able to act in case of a dysbiotic state [132].

2.9.1 Fecal microbiota transplantation as a tool for phage therapy

One of the first studies focusing on the composition of the virome after FMT found the transfer of viral sequences from a healthy donor to pediatric UC patients. Among the sequences, the members of Siphoviridae were transferred with greater efficiency than other groups [136]. Of particular importance is also a study by Broecker et al., who found the phage population of a recipient CDI patient after FMT to be very similar to the donor in contrast to the composition of bacteria [137].

The study of Ott and colleagues [138] demonstrated that the administration of sterile donor fecal matter to patients with Clostridium difficile infection, showing the cessation of symptoms. It is suggested that the effect of FMT can be at least partially

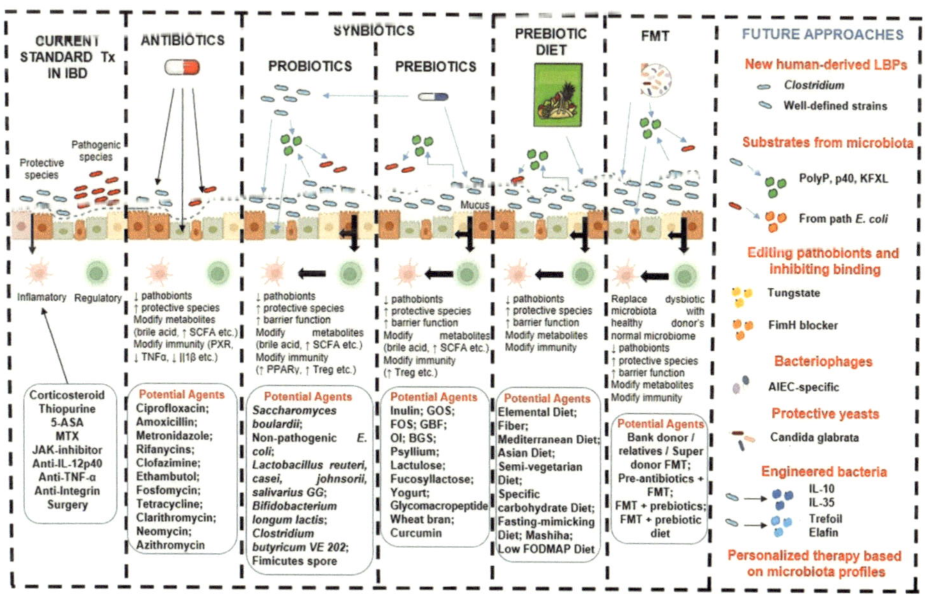

Figure 5.
Schematic overview regarding the status of current standard therapy and microbial-targeted therapies as well as future treatment approaches in IBD. Legend: Tx—therapy; 5-ASA—5-aminosalicylic acid; MTX—methotrexate; JAK—Janus kinase; IL—interleukin; TNF—tumor necrosis factor; SCFA—short chain fatty acid; PXR—pregnane X receptor; PPAR—peroxisome proliferator activated receptor; Treg—regulatory T cell; GOS—galacto-oligosaccharide; FOS—fructo-oligosaccharide; GBF—germinated barley foodstuff; OI—oligofructose-enriched inulin; BGS—bifidogenic growth stimulator; FODMAP—fermentable oligosaccharide; disaccharide, monosaccharide and polyol; FMT—fecal microbiota transplant; LBP—live biotherapeutic product; PolyP—polyphosphate; KFXL—Kangfuxin liquid; path—pathogenic; AIEC—adherent-invasive E. coli.

determined by different parts of the bacterial cell and even non-viable bacterial vectors and phages action.

2.9.2 Safety and efficiency of phage therapy

Galtier et al. [139] infected mice with an adherent-invasive E. coli strain known to be implicated in IBD pathogenesis and administered phage preparation to murine gut sections, living animals, and homogenates of ileal biopsies obtained from CD patients, obtaining a decrease in the colony-forming units of the E. coli strain and a reduction of the clinical picture of dextran sodium sulfate-induced colitis in mice.

Many research studies were not able to find any serious life-threatening adverse effects related to phage treatment [140–142]. A phase I therapy of venous leg ulcers in humans also demonstrated no safety concerns [143]. Another study using transfer of whole viral communities *via* FMT between humans shows that none of the transferred viruses infected human cells [136]. These results highlight the safety of phage therapy, without the development of any serious side effects.

An overview of the current microbial-targeted therapies as well as future treatment approaches for patients with IBD is presented in **Figure 5**.

3. Conclusions: trends toward a personalized treatment in IBD

IBD patients comprise a genetically and clinically heterogeneous population, with particular phenotypes of the disease, severity of the disease, and specific gut microbiota, aspects that lead to different activation of the immune system, response to treatment and disease evolution.

For these reasons, future efforts should be made toward initiation of a personalized treatment in IBD, based on specific evaluation of the gut microbiota and of the profile of the immune system in these patients. This attitude will allow a better understanding of the pathogenesis of IBD and the implementation of specific targeted treatments for the restoration of gut microbiome and correction of bacterial metabolic functions, along with the restoration of the regulatory immune system. In this context, we expect a safer and more efficient therapeutic approach for the management of IBD patients, using novel therapeutic arsenal.

Author details

Daniela Cornelia Lazar[1*], Elena-Alina Moacă[2], Mărioara Cornianu[3], Sorina Tăban[3], Alexandra Faur[4] and Adrian Goldiș[5]

1 Department of Internal Medicine I, University of Medicine and Pharmacy "Victor Babeș" Timișoara, Romania

2 Department of Toxicology, Drug Industry, Management and Legislation, University of Medicine and Pharmacy "Victor Babeș" Timișoara, Romania

3 Department of Pathology, University of Medicine and Pharmacy "Victor Babeș" Timișoara, Romania

4 Department of Anatomy and Embriology, University of Medicine and Pharmacy "Victor Babeș" Timișoara, Romania

5 Department of Gastroenterology, University of Medicine and Pharmacy "Victor Babeș" Timișoara, Romania

*Address all correspondence to: lazar_daniela@yahoo.com

References

[1] Ashton J, Gavin J, Beattie RM. Exclusive enteral nutrition in Crohn's disease: Evidence and practicalities. Clinical Nutrition. 2019;**38**:80-89

[2] Hansen T, Duerksen DR. Enteral nutrition in the management of pediatric and adult Crohn's disease. Nutrients. 2018;**10**:537

[3] Wall C. Use of exclusive enteral nutrition in adults with Crohn's disease: A review. World Journal of Gastroenterology. 2013;**19**:7652-7660

[4] Levine A, Rhodes JM, Lindsay JO, Abreu MT, Kamm MA, Gibson PR, et al. Dietary guidance from the International Organization for the Study of inflammatory bowel diseases. Clinical Gastroenterology and Hepatology. 2020;**18**:1381-1392

[5] Van Rheenen PF, Aloi M, Assa A, Bronsky J, Escher JC, Fagerberg UL, et al. The medical management of paediatric Crohn's Disease: An ECCO-ESPGHAN Guideline Update. Journal of Crohn's & Colitis. 2021;**15**:171-194

[6] Eindor-Abarbanel A, Healey GR, Jacobson K. Therapeutic advances in gut microbiome modulation in patients with inflammatory bowel disease from pediatrics to adulthood. International Journal of Molecular Sciences. 2021;**22**:12506

[7] Lionetti P, Callegari ML, Ferrari S, Cavicchi MC, Pozzi E, De Martino M, et al. Enteral nutrition and microflora in pediatric Crohn's disease. Journal of Parenteral and Enteral Nutrition. 2005;**29**:S173

[8] Quince C, Ijaz UZ, Loman N, Eren AM, Saulnier D, Russell J, et al. Extensive modulation of the fecal metagenome in children with Crohn's disease during exclusive enteral nutrition. The American Journal of Gastroenterology. 2015;**110**:1718-1729

[9] Pigneur B, Lepage P, Mondot S, Schmitz J, Goulet O, Doré J, et al. Mucosal healing and bacterial composition in response to enteral nutrition vs steroid-based induction therapy—A Randomised Prospective Clinical Trial in Children with Crohn's Disease. Journal of Crohn's & Colitis. 2019;**13**:846-855

[10] Costa-Santos MP, Palmela C, Torres J, Ferreira A, Velho S, Ourô S, et al. Preoperative enteral nutrition in adults with complicated Crohn's disease: Effect on disease outcomes and gut microbiota. Nutrients. 2020;**70**:100009

[11] Martyniak A, Medynska-Przeczek A, Wedrychowicz A, Skoczen S, Tomasik PJ. Prebiotics, probiotics, synbiotics, paraprobiotics and postbiotic compounds in IBD. Biomolecules. 2021;**11**:1903

[12] Gibson GR, Hutkins R, Sanders ME, Prescott SE, Reimer RA, Salminen SJ, et al. Expert consensus document: The International Scientific Association for Probiotics and Prebiotics (ISAPP) consensus statement on the definition and scope of prebiotics. Nature Reviews. Gastroenterology & Hepatology. 2017;**14**:491-502

[13] Cummings JH, Macfarlane GT. Gastrointestinal effects of prebiotics. The British Journal of Nutrition. 2002;**87**:S145-S151

[14] Van Loo J. The specificity of the interaction with intestinal bacterial fermentation by prebiotics determines

their physiological efficacy. Nutrition Research Reviews. 2004;**17**:89-98

[15] Benjamin JL, Hedin CR, Koutsoumpas A, Ng SC, McCarthy NE, Hart AL, et al. Randomised, double-blind, placebo-controlled trial of fructo-oligosaccharides in active Crohn's disease. Gut. 2011;**60**:923-929

[16] Manns MP, Bischoff SC. Effect of oral lactulose on clinical and immunohistochemical parameters in patients with inflammatory bowel disease: a pilot study. BMC Gastroenterol. 2007;7:36

[17] Kanauchi O, Mitsuyama K, Homma T, Takahama K, Fujiyama Y, Andoh A, et al. Treatment of ulcerative colitis patients by long-term administration of germinated barley foodstuff: Multi-center open trial. International Journal of Molecular Medicine. 2003;**12**:701-704

[18] Casellas F, Borruel N, Torrejón A, Varela E, Antolin M, Guarner F, et al. Oral oligofructose-enriched inulin supplementation in acute ulcerative colitis is well tolerated and associated with lowered faecal calprotectin. Alimentary Pharmacology & Therapeutics. 2007;**25**:1061-1067

[19] Hanai H, Kanauchi O, Mitsuyama K, Andoh A, Takeuchi K, Takayuki I, et al. Germinated barley foodstuff prolongs remission in patients with ulcerative colitis. International Journal of Molecular Medicine. 2004;**13**:643-647

[20] Hallert C, Kaldma M, Petersson BG. Ispaghula husk may relieve gastrointestinal symptoms in ulcerative colitis in remission. Scandinavian Journal of Gastroenterology. 1991;**26**:747-750

[21] Fernández-Bañares F, Hinojosa J, Sánchez-Lombraña JL, Navarro E, Martínez-Salmerón JF, García-Pugés A, et al. Randomized clinical trial of Plantago ovata seeds (dietary fiber) as compared with mesalamine in maintaining remission in ulcerative colitis. Spanish Group for the Study of Crohn's Disease and Ulcerative Colitis (GETECCU). The American Journal of Gastroenterology. 1999;**94**:427-433

[22] Azad MAK, Sarker M, Li T, Yin J. Probiotic species in the modulation of gut microbiota: An overview. BioMed Research International. 2018;**2018**:9478630

[23] Yoshimatsu Y, Mikami Y, Kanai T. Bacteriotherapy for inflammatory bowel disease. Inflammation and Regeneration. 2021;**41**:3

[24] Tamaki H, Nakase H, Inoue S, Kawanami C, Itani T, Ohana M, et al. Efficacy of probiotic treatment with Bifidobacterium longum 536 for induction of remission in active ulcerative colitis: A randomized, double-blinded, placebo-controlled multicenter trial. Digestive Endoscopy. 2016;**28**:67-74

[25] De Vrese M, Schrezenmeir J. Probiotics, prebiotics, and synbiotics. Advances in Biochemical Engineering/Biotechnology. 2008;**111**:1-66

[26] Martín R, Miquel S, Ulmer J, Kechaou N, Langella P, Bermúdez-Humarán LG. Role of commensal and probiotic bacteria in human health: A focus on inflammatory bowel disease. Microbial Cell Factories. 2013;**12**:71

[27] Abraham BP, Quigley EMM. Probiotics in inflammatory bowel disease. Gastroenterology Clinics of North America. 2017;**46**:769-782

[28] Ghavami SB, Yadegar A, Aghdaei HA, Sorrentino D, Farmani M, Mir AS, et al. Immunomodulation and

generation of tolerogenic dendritic cells by probiotic bacteria in patients with inflammatory bowel disease. International Journal of Molecular Science. 2020;**21**:6266

[29] Jakubczyk D, Leszczynska K, Górska S. The effectiveness of probiotics in the treatment of inflammatory bowel disease (IBD): A critical review. Nutrients. 2020;**12**:1973

[30] Ekmekciu I, Von Klitzing E, Fiebiger U, Neumann C, Bacher P, Scheffold A, et al. The probiotic compound VSL#3 modulates mucosal, peripheral, and systemic immunity following murine broad-spectrum antibiotic treatment. Frontiers in Cellular and Infection Microbiology. 2017;**7**:1-19

[31] Zoppi G, Cinquetti M, Benini A, Bonamini E, Minelli EB. Modulation of the intestinal ecosystem by probiotics and lactulose in children during treatment with ceftriaxone. Current Therapeutic Research, Clinical and Experimental. 2001;**62**:418-435

[32] Wang L, Guo MJ, Gao Q, Yang JF, Yang L, Pang XL, et al. The effects of probiotics on total cholesterol. Medicine (United States). 2018;**97**:e9679

[33] Reid G, Bruce AW, Fraser N, Heinemann C, Owen J, Henning B. Oral probiotics can resolve urogenital infections. FEMS Immunology and Medical Microbiology. 2001;**30**:49-52

[34] Yoshimatsu Y, Yamada A, Furukawa R, Sono K, Osamura A, Nakamura K, et al. Effectiveness of probiotic therapy for the prevention of relapse in patients with inactive ulcerative colitis. World Journal of Gastroenterology. 2015;**21**:5985-5994

[35] Yılmaz I, Dolar ME, Özpınar H. Effect of administering kefir on the changes in fecal microbiota and symptoms of inflammatory bowel disease: A randomized controlled trial. The Turkish Journal of Gastroenterology. 2019;**30**:242-253

[36] Shadnoush M, Hosseini RS, Khalilnezhad A, Navai L, Goudarzi H, Vaezjalali M. Effects of probiotics on gut microbiota in patients with inflammatory bowel disease: A double-blind, Placebo-controlled Clinical Trial. Korean Journal of Gastroenterology. 2015;**65**:215-221

[37] Palumbo VD, Romeo M, Marino Gammazza A, Carini F, Damiani P, Damiano G, et al. The long-term effects of probiotics in the therapy of ulcerative colitis: A clinical study. Biomedical Paper Medicine Faculty University. 2016;**160**:372-377

[38] Fan H, Du J, Liu X, Zheng WW, Zhuang ZH, Wang CD, et al. Effects of pentasa-combined probiotics on the microflora structure and prognosis of patients with inflammatory bowel disease. The Turkish Journal of Gastroenterology. 2019;**30**:680-685

[39] Su H, Kang Q, Wang H, Yin H, Duan L, Liu Y, et al. Effects of glucocorticoids combined with probiotics in treating Crohn's disease on inflammatory factors and intestinal microflora. Experimental and Therapeutic Medicine. 2018;**16**:2999-3003

[40] Bjarnason I, Sission G, Hayee B. A randomised, double-blind, placebo-controlled trial of a multi-strain probiotic in patients with asymptomatic ulcerative colitis and Crohn's disease. Inflammopharmacology. 2019;**27**:465-473

[41] Fedorak RN, Feagan BG, Hotte N, Leddin D, Dieleman LA, Petrunia DM, et al. The probiotic VSL#3 has anti-inflammatory effects and could reduce

endoscopic recurrence after surgery for Crohn's disease. Clinical Gastroenterology and Hepatology. 2015;**13**:928-935

[42] Matsuoka K, Uemura Y, Kanai T, Kunisaki R, Suzuki Y, Yokoyama K, et al. Efficacy of Bifidobacterium breve fermented milk in maintaining remission of ulcerative colitis. Digestive Diseases and Sciences. 2018;**63**:1910-1919

[43] Astó E, Méndez I, Audivert S, Farran-Codina A, Espadaler J. The efficacy of probiotics, prebiotic inulin-type fructans, and synbiotics in human ulcerative colitis: A systematic review and meta-analysis. Nutrients. 2019;**11**:293

[44] Zhang XF, Guan XX, Tang YJ, Sun JF, Wang XK, Wang WD, et al. Clinical effects and gut microbiota changes of using probiotics, prebiotics or synbiotics in inflammatory bowel disease: A systematic review and meta-analysis. European Journal of Nutrition. 2021;**60**:2855

[45] Jia K, Tong X, Wang R, Song X. The clinical effects of probiotics for inflammatory bowel disease: A meta-analysis. Medicine. 2018;**97**:e13792

[46] Puvvada SR, Luvsannyam E, Patel D, Hassan Z, Hamid P. Probiotics in inflammatory bowel disease: Are we back to square one? Cureus. 2020;**12**:e10247

[47] Dore MP, Bibbò S, Fresi G, Bassotti G, Pes GM. Side effects associated with probiotic use in adult patients with inflammatory bowel disease: A systematic review and meta-analysis of randomized controlled trials. Nutrients. 2019;**11**:2913

[48] Dore MP, Rocchi C, Longo NP, Scanu AM, Vidili G, Padedda F, et al. Effect of probiotic use on adverse events in adult patients with inflammatory bowel disease: A Retrospective Cohort Study. Probiotics Antimicrobial Proteins. 2020;**12**:152-159

[49] Mishra J, Stubbs M, Kuang L, Vara N, Kumar P, Kumar N. Inflammatory bowel disease therapeutics: A focus on probiotic engineering. Mediators of Inflammation Volume. 2022;**962**:15

[50] Glassner KL, Abraham BP, Quigley EMM. The microbiome and inflammatory bowel disease. The Journal of Allergy and Clinical Immunology. 2020s;**145**:16-27

[51] Goh YJ, Barrangou R. Harnessing CRISPR-Cas systems for precision engineering of designer probiotic lactobacilli. Current Opinion in Biotechnology. 2019;**56**:163-171

[52] Hamady ZZ, Scott N, Farrar MD, et al. Xylan-regulated delivery of human keratinocyte growth factor-2 to the inflamed colon by the human anaerobic commensal bacterium Bacteroides ovatus. Gut. 2010;**59**(4):461-469

[53] Del Carmen S, De Leblanc AD, Perdigon G, et al. Evaluation of the anti-inflammatory effect of milk fermented by a strain of IL-10-producing Lactococcus lactis using a murine model of Crohn's disease. Journal of Molecular Microbiology and Biotechnology. 2011;**21**:138-146

[54] Steidler L, Hans W, Schotte L, et al. Treatment of murine colitis by Lactococcus lactis Secreting interleukin-10. Science. 2000;**289**(5483):1352-1355

[55] Veenbergen S, Li P, Raatgeep HC, et al. IL-10 signaling in dendritic cells controls IL-1β-mediated IFNγ secretion by human CD4+ T cells: Relevance to

inflammatory bowel disease. Mucosal Immunology. 2019;**12**(5):1201-1211

[56] Friedrich M, Pohin M, Powrie F. Cytokine networks in the pathophysiology of inflammatory bowel disease. Immunity. 2019;**50**:992-1006

[57] Barra M, Danino T, Garrido D. Engineered probiotics for detection and treatment of inflammatory intestinal diseases. Frontiers in Bioengineering and Biotechnology. 2020;**8**:265

[58] Lavasani S, Dzhambazov B, Nouri M, et al. A novel probiotic mixture exerts a therapeutic effect on experimental autoimmune encephalomyelitis mediated by IL-10 producing regulatory T cells. PLoS One. 2010;**5**:e9009

[59] Andrews C, McLean MH, Durum SK. Interleukin-27 as a novel therapy for inflammatory bowel disease: A critical review of the literature. Inflammatory Bowel Diseases. 2016;**22**:2255-2264

[60] McLean MH, Andrews C, Hanson ML, et al. Interleukin-27 is a potential rescue therapy for acute severe colitis through interleukin-10-dependent, T-cell-independent attenuation of colonic mucosal innate immune responses. Inflammatory Bowel Diseases. 2017;**23**:1983-1995

[61] Hanson ML, Hixon JA, Li W, et al. Oral delivery of IL-27 recombinant bacteria attenuates immune colitis in mice. Gastroenterology. 2014;**146**:210-221

[62] Al-Meghaiseeb ES, Al-Robayan AA, Al-Otaibi MM, Arfin M, Al-Asmari AK. Association of tumor necrosis factor-alpha and -beta gene polymorphisms in inflammatory bowel disease. Journal of Inflammation Research. 2016;**9**:133-140

[63] Holmgren J, Czerkinsky C. Mucosal immunity and vaccines. Nature Medicine. 2005;**11**:S45-S53

[64] Jiang B, Li Z, Ou B, Duan Q, Zhu G. Targeting ideal oral vaccine vectors based on probiotics: A systematical view. Applied Microbiology and Biotechnology. 2019;**103**:3941-3953

[65] Isolauri E, Majamaa H, Arvola T, Rantala I, Virtanen E, Arvilommi H. Lactobacillus casei strain GG reverses increased intestinal permeability induced by cow milk insuckling rats. Gastroenterology. 1993;**105**:1643-1650

[66] Mathipa MG, Thantsha MS. Probiotic engineering: Towards development of robust probiotic strains with enhanced functional properties and for targeted control of enteric pathogens. Gut Pathogens. 2017;**9**:28

[67] Akutko K, Stawarski A. Probiotics, prebiotics and synbiotics in inflammatory bowel diseases. Journal of Clinical Medicine. 2021;**10**:2466

[68] Wasilewski A, Zielinska M, Storr M, Fichna J. Beneficial effects of probiotics, prebiotics, synbiotics, and psychobiotics in inflammatory bowel disease. Inflammatory Bowel Diseases. 2015;**21**:1674-1682

[69] Steed H, Macfarlane GT, Blackett KL, Bahrami B, Reynolds N, Walsh SV, et al. Clinical trial: The microbiological and immunological effects of synbiotic consumption—A randomized double-blind placebo-controlled study in active Crohn's disease. Alimentary Pharmacology & Therapeutics. 2010;**32**:872-883

[70] Furrie E, Macfarlane S, Kennedy A, Cummings JH, Walsh SV, O'neil DA, et al. Synbiotic therapy (Bifidobacterium longum/Synergy 1) initiates resolution of inflammation in patients with active ulcerative colitis: A randomised controlled pilot trial. Gut. 2005;**54**:242-249

[71] Chermesh I, Tamir A, Reshef R, Chowers Y, Suissa A, Katz D, et al. Failure of Synbiotic 2000 to prevent postoperative recurrence of Crohn's disease. Digestive Diseases and Sciences. 2007;**52**:385-389

[72] Fujimori S, Gudis K, Mitsui K, Seo T, Yonezawa M, Tanaka S, et al. A randomized controlled trial on the efficacy of synbiotic versus probiotic or prebiotic treatment to improve the quality of life in patients with ulcerative colitis. Nutrition. 2009;**25**:520-525

[73] Ishikawa H, Matsumoto S, Ohashi Y, Imaoka A, Setoyama H, Umesaki Y, et al. Beneficial effects of probiotic bifidobacterium and galacto-oligosaccharide in patients with ulcerative colitis: A randomized controlled study. Digestion. 2011;**84**:128-133

[74] Floch MH. Probiotic Safety and Risk Factors. Journal of Clinical Gastroenterology. 2013;**47**:375-376

[75] Vahabnezhad E, Mochon AB, Wozniak LJ, Ziring DA. Lactobacillus bacteremia associated with probiotic use in a pediatric patient with ulcerative colitis. Journal of Clinical Gastroenterology. 2013;**47**:437-439

[76] Martín R, Langella P. Emerging health concepts in the probiotics field: Streamlining the definitions. Frontiers in Microbiology. 2019;**10**:1047

[77] De Almada CN, de Almada CN, de Sant'Ana AS. Paraprobiotics as potential agents for improving animal health. In: Probiotics and Prebiotics in Animal Health and Food Safety. Berlin/Heidelberg, Germany: Springer International Publishing; 2018. pp. 247-268

[78] Akter S, Jung J-HP, Jung HK. Potential health-promoting benefits of paraprobiotics, inactivated probiotic cells. Journal of Microbiology Biotechnology. 2020;**30**:477-481

[79] De Almada CN, Almada CN, Martinez RCR, Sant'Ana AS. Paraprobiotics: Evidences on their ability to modify biological responses, inactivation methods and perspectives on their application in foods. Trends in Food Science and Technology. 2016;**58**:96-114

[80] Barros CP, Guimarães JT, Esmerino EA, Duarte MCK, Silva MC, Silva R, et al. Paraprobiotics and postbiotics: Concepts and potential applications in dairy products. Current Opinion in Food Science. 2020;**32**:1-8

[81] Sharma M, Shukla G. Metabiotics: One step ahead of probiotics; an insight into mechanisms involved in anticancerous effect in colorectal cancer. Frontiers in Microbiology. 2016;**7**:1940

[82] Fang SB, Shih HY, Huang CH, Li LT, Chen CC, Fang HW. Live and heat-killed Lactobacillus rhamnosus GG upregulate gene expression of pro-inflammatory cytokines in 5-fluorouracil-pretreated Caco-2 cells. Supportive Care in Cancer. 2014;**22**:1647-1654

[83] Ryu YH, Baik JE, Yang JS, Kang SS, Im J, Yun CH, et al. Differential immunostimulatory effects of gram-positive bacteria due to their lipoteichoic acids. International Immunopharmacology. 2009;**9**:127-133

[84] Teame T, Wang A, Xie M, Zhang Z, Yang Y, Ding Q, et al. Paraprobiotics and postbiotics of probiotic lactobacilli, their positive effects on the host and action mechanisms: A review. Frontiers in Nutrition. 2020;**7**:570344

[85] Shenderov BA. Metabiotics: Novel idea or natural development of probiotic

conception. Microbial Ecology in Health and Disease. 2013;**24**

[86] Oleskin AV, Shenderov BA. Microbial Communication and Microbiota-Host Interactivity: Neurophysiological, Biotechnological, and Biopolitical Implications. Hauppauge, NY, USA: Nova Science Publishers; 2020

[87] Macfarlane S, Macfarlane GT. Regulation of short-chain fatty acid production. The Proceedings of the Nutrition Society. 2003;**62**:67-72

[88] Russo E, Giudici F, Fiorindi C, Ficari F, Scaringi S, Amedei A. Immunomodulating activity and therapeutic effects of short chain fatty acids and tryptophan post-biotics in inflammatory bowel disease. Frontiers in Immunology. 2019;**10**:2754

[89] Topping DL, Clifton PM. Short-chain fatty acids and human colonic function: Roles of resistant starch and nonstarch polysaccharides. Physiological Reviews. 2001;**81**:1031-1064

[90] Poul EL, Loison C, Struyf S, Springael J-Y, Lannoy V, Decobecq M-E, et al. Functional characterization of human receptors for short chain fatty acids and their role in polymorphonuclear cell activation. The Journal of Biological Chemistry. 2003;**278**:25481-25489

[91] Canani RB, di Costanzo M, Leone L, Pedata M, Meli R, Calignano A. Potential beneficial effects of butyrate in intestinal and extraintestinal diseases. World Journal of Gastroenterology. 2011;**17**:1519-1528

[92] Scheppach W, Weiler F. The butyrate story: Old wine in new bottles? Current Opinion in Clinical Nutrition and Metabolic Care. 2004;**7**:563-567

[93] Brummer R-JM. Effect of butyrate enemas on inflammation and antioxidant status in the colonic mucosa of patients with ulcerative colitis in remission. Clinical Nutrition. 2010;**29**:738-744

[94] Vernia P, Annese V, Bresci G, D'Albasio G, D'Incà R, Giaccari S, et al. Topical butyrate improves efficacy of 5-ASA in refractory distal ulcerative colitis: Results of a Multicentre Trial. European Journal of Clinical Investigation. 2003;**33**:244-248

[95] Di Sabatino A, Morera R, Ciccocioppo R, Cazzola P, Gotti S, Tinozzi FP, et al. Oral butyrate for mildly to moderately active Crohn's disease. Alimentary Pharmacology & Therapeutics. 2005;**22**:789-794

[96] Matsumoto N, Riley S, Fraser D, Al-Assaf S, Ishimura E, Wolever T, et al. Butyrate modulates TGF-B1 generation and function: Potential renal benefit for Acacia (Sen) supergumtm (Gum Arabic)? Kidney International. 2006;**69**:257-265

[97] Wanders D, Graff EC, Judd RL. Effects of high fat diet on GPR109A and GPR81 gene expression. Biochemical and Biophysical Research Communications. 2012;**425**:278-283

[98] Singh N, Gurav A, Sivaprakasam S, Brady E, Padia R, Shi H, et al. Activation of Gpr109a, receptor for niacin and the commensal metabolite butyrate. Suppresses Colonic Inflammation and Carcinogenesis. Immunity. 2014;**40**:128-139

[99] Al-Lahham SH, Peppelenbosch MP, Roelofsen H, Vonk RJ, Venema K. Biological effects of propionic acid in humans; Metabolism, potential applications and underlying mechanisms. Biochimica Biophysica Acta. 1801;**2010**:1175-1183

[100] Tedelind S, Westberg F, Kjerrulf M, Vidal A. Anti-inflammatory properties of the short-chain fatty acids acetate and propionate: A study with relevance to inflammatory bowel disease. World Journal of Gastroenterology. 2007;**13**:2826-2832

[101] Perry RJ, Peng L, Barry NA, Cline GW, Zhang D, Cardone RL, et al. Acetate mediates a microbiome–brain–β-cell axis to promote metabolic syndrome. Nature. 2016;**534**:213-217

[102] Macia L, Tan J, Vieira AT, Leach K, Stanley D, Luong S, et al. Metabolite-sensing receptors GPR43 and GPR109A facilitate dietary fibre-induced gut homeostasis through regulation of the inflammasome. Nature Communications. 2015;**6**:1-15

[103] Vernia P, Marcheggiano A, Caprilli R, Frieri G, Corrao G, Valpiani D, et al. Short-chain fatty acid topical treatment in distal ulcerative colitis. Alimentary Pharmacology & Therapeutics. 1995;**9**:309-313

[104] Lührs H, Gerke T, Müller JG, Melcher R, Schauber J, Boxberger F, et al. Butyrate inhibits NF-KB activation in lamina propria macrophages of patients with ulcerative colitis. Scandinavian Journal of Gastroenterology. 2002:458-466

[105] Senagore AJ, MacKeigan JM, Scheider M, Ebrom JS. Short-chain fatty acid enemas: A cost-effective alternative in the treatment of nonspecific proctosigmoiditis. Diseases of the Colon and Rectum. 1992;**35**:923-927

[106] Scheppach W, Sommer H, Kirchner T, Paganelli G-M, Bartram P, Christl S, et al. Effect of butyrate enemas on the colonic mucosa in distal ulcerative colitis. Gastroenterology. 1992;**103**:51-56

[107] Scheppach W. Treatment of distal ulcerative colitis with short-chain fatty acid enemas. A Placebo-Controlled Trial.German Austrian SCFA Study Group. Digestive Disease Science. 1996;**41**:2254-2259

[108] Steinhart AH, Hiruki T, Brzezinski A, Baker JP. Treatment of left-sided ulcerative colitis with butyrate enemas: A Controlled Trial. Alimentary Pharmacology & Therapeutics. 1996;**10**:729-736

[109] Breuer RI, Soergel KH, Lashner BA, Christ ML, Hanauer SB, Vanagunas A, et al. Short chain fatty acid rectal irrigation for left-sided ulcerative colitis: A Randomised, Placebo Controlled Trial. Gut. 1997;**40**:485

[110] Schiering C, Wincent E, Metidji A, Iseppon A, Li Y, Potocnik AJ, et al. Feedback control of AHR signalling regulates intestinal immunity. Nature. 2017;**542**:242-245

[111] Levin AD, van den Brink GR. Selective inhibition of mucosal serotonin as treatment for IBD? Gut. 2014;**63**:866-867

[112] Gao J, Xu K, Liu H, Liu G, Bai M, Peng C, et al. Impact of the gut microbiota on intestinal immunity mediated by tryptophan metabolism. Frontiers in Cellular and Infection Microbiology. 2018;**8**:13

[113] Nikolaus S, Schulte B, Al-Massad N, Thieme F, Schulte DM, Bethge J, et al. Increased tryptophan metabolism is associated with activity of inflammatory bowel diseases. Gastroenterology. 2017;**153**:1504-1516

[114] Wolf AM, Wolf D, Rumpold H, Moschen AR, Kaser A, Obrist P, et al. Overexpression of indoleamine 2,3-dioxygenase in human inflammatory

bowel disease. Clinical Immunology. 2004;**113**:47-55

[115] Lamas B, Richard ML, Leducq V, Pham H-P, Michel M-L, da Costa G, et al. CARD9 impacts colitis by altering gut microbiota metabolism of tryptophan into aryl hydrocarbon receptor ligands. Nature Medicine. 2016;**22**:598-605

[116] Cervantes-Barragan L, Chai JN, Tianero MD, di Luccia B, Ahern PP, Merriman J, et al. Lactobacillus Reuteri induces gut intraepithelial CD4+CD8αα+ T Cells. Science. 2017;**357**:806-810

[117] Lee J-Y, Cevallos SA, Byndloss MX, Tiffany CR, Olsan EE, Butler BP, et al. High-fat diet and antibiotics cooperatively impair mitochondrial bioenergetics to trigger dysbiosis that exacerbates pre-inflammatory bowel disease. Cell Host Microbe. 2020;**28**:273-284

[118] Oka A, Sartor RB. Microbial-based and microbial-targeted therapies for inflammatory bowel diseases. Digestive Diseases and Sciences. 2020;**65**:757-788

[119] Maccaferri S, Vitali B, Klinder A, Kolida S, Ndagijimana M, Laghi L, et al. Rifaximin modulates the colonic microbiota of patients with Crohn's disease: An in vitro approach using a continuous culture colonic model system. The Journal of Antimicrobial Chemotherapy. 2010;**65**:2556-2565

[120] Bücker R, Schulz E, Günzel D, Bojarski C, Lee I-FM, John LJ, et al. α-Haemolysin of Escherichia coliin IBD: A potentiator of inflammatory activity in the colon. Gut. 2014;**63**:1893-1901

[121] Lev-Tzion R, Ledder O, Shteyer E, Tan MLN, Uhlig HH, Turner D. Oral vancomycin and gentamicin for treatment of very early onset inflammatory bowel disease. Digestion. 2017;**95**:310-313

[122] Townsend CM, Parker CE, MacDonald JK, Nguyen TM, Jairath V, Feagan BG, et al. Antibiotics for induction and maintenance of remission in Crohn's disease. Cochrane Database of Systematic Reviews. 2019;**2**:CD012

[123] Sprockett D, Fischer N, Boneh RS, Turner D, Kierkus J, Sladek M, et al. Treatment-specific composition of the gut microbiota is associated with disease remission in a pediatric Crohn's disease Cohort. Inflammatory Bowel Diseases. 2019;**25**:1927-1938

[124] Zhang L, Ma X, Liu P, Ge W, Hu L, Zuo Z, et al. Treatment and mechanism of fecal microbiota transplantation in mice with experimentally induced ulcerative colitis. Experimental Biology and Medicine (Maywood, N.J.). 2021;**246**(13):1563-1575

[125] Imdad A, Nicholson MR, Tanner-Smith EE, Zackular JP, Gomez-Duarte OG, Beaulieu DB, et al. Fecal transplantation for treatment of inflammatory bowel disease. Cochrane Database of Systematic Reviews. 2018;**11**:CD012

[126] Fang H, Fu L, Wang J. Protocol for fecal microbiota transplantation in inflammatory bowel disease: A systematic review and meta-analysis. BioMed Research International. 2018;**894**:11

[127] Sokol H, Landman C, Seksik P, et al. Fecal microbiota transplantation to maintain remission in Crohn's disease: A pilot randomized controlled study. Microbiome. 2020;**8**:12

[128] Santiago-Rodriguez T, Hollister E. Human virome and disease: High-throughput sequencing for virus

discovery, identification of phage-bacteria dysbiosis and development of therapeutic approaches with emphasis on the human gut. Viruses. 2019;**11**:656

[129] Pérez-Brocal V, García-López R, Nos P, Beltrán B, Moret I, Moya A. Metagenomic analysis of Crohn's disease patients identifies changes in the virome and microbiome related to disease status and therapy, and detects potential interactions and biomarkers. Inflammatory Bowel Diseases. 2015;**21**:2515-2532

[130] Fernandes MA, Verstraete SG, Phan TG, Deng X, Stekol E, LaMere B, et al. Enteric virome and bacterial microbiota in children with ulcerative colitis and Crohn Disease. Journal of Pediatric Gastroenterology and Nutrition. 2019;**68**:30-36

[131] Duerkop BA, Kleiner M, Paez-Espino D, Zhu W, Bushnell B, Hassell B, et al. Murine colitis reveals a disease-associated bacteriophage community. Nature Microbiology. 2018;**3**:11023-11031

[132] Maronek M, Link R, Ambro L, Gardlik R. Phages and their role in gastrointestinal disease: Focus on inflammatory bowel disease. Cell. 2020;**9**:1013

[133] Zhang L, Hou X, Sun L, He T, Wei R, Pang M, et al. Corrigendum: *Staphylococcus aureus* bacteriophage suppresses LPS-induced inflammation in MAC-T bovine mammary epithelial cells. Frontiers in Microbiology. 2018;**9**:3389

[134] Górski A, Bollyky PL, Przybylski M, Borysowski J, Miedzybrodzki R, Jonczyk-Matysiak E, et al. Perspectives of phage therapy in non-bacterial infections. Frontiers in Microbiology. 2019;**9**:1

[135] Lemire S, Yehl KM, Lu TK. Phage-based applications in synthetic biology. Annual Review in Virology. 2018;**5**:453-476

[136] Chehoud C, Dryga A, Hwang Y, Nagy-Szakal D, Hollister EB, Luna RA, et al. Transfer of viral communities between human individuals during fecal microbiota transplantation. mBio. 2016;**7**:1-8

[137] Broecker F, Russo G, Klumpp J, Moelling K. Stable core virome despite variable microbiome after fecal transfer. Gut Microbes. 2017;**8**:214-220

[138] Ott SJ, Waetzig GH, Rehman A, Moltzau-Anderson J, Bharti R, Grasis JA, et al. Efficacy of sterile fecal filtrate transfer for treating patients with clostridium difficile infection. Gastroenterology. 2017;**152**:799-811

[139] Galtier MA. Bacteriophages targeting adherent invasive Escherichia coli strains as a promising new treatment for Crohn's disease. Journal of Crohn's & Colitis. 2017;**11**:840-847

[140] Speck P, Smithyman A. Safety and efficacy of phage therapy via the intravenous route. FEMS Microbiology Letters. 2016;**363**:1-6

[141] Malik DJ, Sokolov IJ, Vinner GK, Mancuso F, Cinquerrui S, Vladisavljevic GT, et al. Formulation, stabilisation and encapsulation of bacteriophage for phage therapy. Advances in Colloid and Interface Science. 2017;**249**:100-133

[142] McCallin S, Sarker SA, Sultana S, Oechslin F, Brssow H. Metagenome analysis of Russian and Georgian Pyophage cocktails and a placebo-controlled safety trial of single phage versus phage cocktail in healthy Staphylococcus aureus carriers.

Environmental Microbiology. 2018;**20**:3278-3293

[143] Rhoads DD, Wolcott RD, Kuskowski MA, Wolcott BM, Ward LS, Sulakvelidze A. Bacteriophage therapy of venous leg ulcers in humans: Results of a phase I safety trial. Journal of Wound Care. 2009;**18**:237-243

Chapter 5

Drug-Related Enteropathy

Octavio Gómez-Escudero

Abstract

Over 700 drugs have been implicated as cause of chronic diarrhea and potential enteral damage. Pathophysiologic mechanisms include intrinsic malabsorption as their main mode of action (i.e., acarbose or orlistat), increased risk of microscopic colitis/enteritis (proton-pump inhibitors (PPI), non-steroidal anti-inflammatory drugs (NSAID), selective serotonin reuptake inhibitors (SSRI)), dysbiosis (antibiotics, metformin, PPI), and microscopic or overt enteropathy (angiotensin inhibitors, antineoplastic agents, targeted therapy and check-point inhibitors). According to type, diarrhea can be malabsorptive, inflammatory or mixed, and may affect different portions of small intestine, colon, or both. Drug-induced enteropathy ranges from asymptomatic histological changes to macroscopic damage similar to that seen in inflammatory bowel disease. Treatment may include discontinuation of drug, correction of dysbiosis, and in severe cases, directed therapy towards intestinal wall inflammatory states, in similar mode as in other inflammatory bowel diseases.

Keywords: drugs, medications, chronic diarrhea, enteropathy, malabsorption, side-effect, bowel inflammation

1. Introduction

Diarrhea is one of the most common symptoms in the gastroenterologist clinical practice. It is defined as an increase in the average number of bowel movements, stool output and/or weight, or a reduced stool consistency, and according to duration, can be acute if it lasts less than 7 days, persistent acute (>7 days and < 14 days), sub-acute (>14 days and < 28 days), or chronic (>4 weeks) [1–6]. Most episodes of acute diarrhea occur as a result of infectious agents or dietary transgression. Acute persistent and subacute diarrhea may be caused by unidentified microorganisms or might be secondary to medications [1]. Chronic diarrhea is one of those conditions with the broadest differential diagnosis, that includes anatomical and/or physiologic abnormalities of the gastrointestinal (GI) tract, inflammatory or neoplastic conditions, malabsorptive disorders, drug side effects, dysbiosis, functional as well as post-infectious syndromes such as small intestine bowel overgrowth (SIBO), functional diarrhea or post-infectious irritable bowel syndrome (Pi-IBS) [2–6]. One of the most common, albeit rarely unconsidered causes, is drug-side effect [7, 8]. A large number of at least 700 drugs have been implicated as cause of chronic diarrhea through a number of different, and sometimes overlapped pathophysiologic mechanisms [9]. Although initial therapy is drug withdrawal, in several cases treatment directed at pathophysiologic mechanism is needed to revert damage and improve symptoms.

2. Mechanisms of enteral damage

Enteral damage and consequent symptoms such as diarrhea, bloating, flatulence and pain may be mediated through different mechanisms falling into two main categories: (1) Functional damage: it can be caused by abnormalities in any of the mechanisms involving digestion (maldigestion) and/or absorption (malabsorption), GI motility disturbances, alterations in the water and electrolyte absorption and/or secretion mechanisms, and altered microbiota and/or microbiome (dysbiosis), and (2) Microscopic or overt mucosal damage: this can be caused by direct contact of the drug, ischemic-related damage, systemic inflammatory or autoimmune mechanisms, and may affect different portions of the small intestine, colon, or both (**Figure 1**, [9]). According to the involved mechanism, main symptoms may predominate diarrhea, malabsorptive complaints such as steatorrhea, weight loss and anemia, or abdominal pain, and in severe cases, occult or overt bleeding.

3. Maldigestion and malabsorption

Small intestine is involved in both digestive and absorptive processes of all major nutrients, fatty acids and multiple ions, occurring across the entire intestinal wall at different levels. Normal functional anatomy includes a full bowel length, normal intestinal villi and absorptive capacity, conserved neuroendocrine regulatory systems, and a normal motility activity, particularly the major motor complex (MMC) [10]. Several drugs may interfere with one or multiple mechanisms associated with either digestion processes or mechanisms associated with intestinal absorption. Alpha-glucosidase inhibitors such as acarbose decrease carbohydrate digestion, lipase-inhibitors such as orlistat and cetilistat affect fat absorption, bile acid binding resins such as cholestyramine or colestipol affects not only bile acid absorption but also that

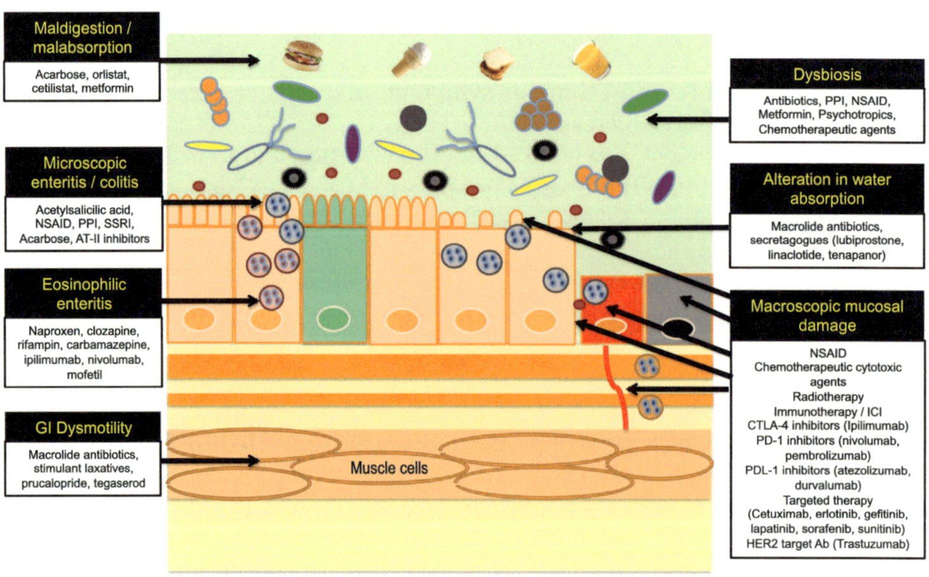

Figure 1.
Pathophysiologic mechanisms of enteropathy according to drug type.

of vitamin B12 and lipid-soluble vitamins, but as they are used in bile-acid diarrhea as main therapeutic indication, they can be associated with constipation instead of diarrhea. Different drugs may induce calcium precipitation, such as aluminum or tetracycline, with further changes in bowel habit. Structural damage leading to villous inflammation and/or atrophy is described in the mucosal damage section [11].

3.1 Drugs associated with interference in digestion and/or malabsorption processes

A number of drugs used to treat metabolic conditions such as diabetes mellitus and obesity have intrinsic malabsorptive mechanisms as their main mode of action, and may lead to diarrhea and other related symptoms due to those mechanisms.

Acarbose is a pseudo-tetrasaccharide that selectively inhibits alpha-glucosidase activity in the brush border membrane of the small intestine, an essential enzyme for digestion of starch, maltose and sucrose, delaying glucose absorption from carbohydrate food and thus improving glycemic control among patients with either glucose intolerance or diabetes mellitus [12]. Among common side effects, mainly intrinsic to its mode of action, include flatulence, bloating and diarrhea [13].

Orlistat is a reversible inhibitor of gastric and pancreatic lipoprotein lipases, resulting in inhibition of up to 30% of dietary fat absorption, decreasing fat mass, as well as levels of the regulatory hormone leptin as patients lose weight [14]. Most common adverse events, also intrinsic to its mechanism of action, are diarrhea, steatorrhea, flatulence, bloating and abdominal pain [15]. Recently a second lipase inhibitor, cetilistat, has shown similar efficacy with fewer side effects when compared to orlistat, however prevalence of diarrhea may be as high as 25% of users [16].

Metformin, a dimethyl-biguanide, is an oral glucose-lowering agent absorbed in the small intestine, that has several modes of action: it reduces hepatic glucose production by inhibition of hepatic gluconeogenesis, it increases insulin sensitization by increasing plasma glucagon-like-protein (GLP) type 1 concentrations, with a smaller effect on dipeptidyl-peptidase 4 (DPP-4), resulting in increased glucose uptake in the small intestine [17]. It may also induce alterations in enteral microbiome, particularly increased abundance of *Akkermansia muciniphila*, a bacterium reported to improve glucose tolerance by increasing endocannabinoids, reducing inflammation, and increasing gut mucous barrier thickness [18]. Despite these beneficial effects, metformin is frequently associated with GI side effects such as flatulence, bloating, dyspepsia, and diarrhea. A number of potential mechanisms of GI intolerance have been described, including altered transport of serotonin, histamine or both, increased enterocyte lactate concentration, dysbiosis, increased bile acid pool in the distal ileum, bile acid receptor activation, and increased conversion from primary to secondary bile acids, which are pro-secretory, leading to increased water and electrolyte luminal secretion. Most of these side effects are dose-related and decrease with time, or after probiotic use, but may persist or even develop after withdrawal [19].

4. Alterations in motility and water absorption/secretion

As previously mentioned, small intestine is both an absorptive and secretory organ, and most of the water and electrolyte handling in the GI tract is regulated at this level by autonomic nerve system as well as by neuromuscular signal pathways [10]. A number of drugs may alter one or several of the mechanisms associated with normal GI motility and/or water and electrolyte secretion including laxatives, motilin analog antibiotics, enterokinetic drugs, secretagogues, colchicine, and prostaglandin analogs.

4.1 Drugs associated with diarrhea due to dysmotility and/or alterations in water absorption and/or secretion

Several antibiotics, particularly the macrolides (e.g., azithromycin, clarithromycin, erythromycin), act as motilin analogues. Motilin is a hormone that induces MMC activity though four distinct phases: first one is a period of near quiescence, second is characterized by irregular small-amplitude waves, phase III induces high-amplitude propulsive contractions all along the small intestine, and during phase IV, motor activity declines to basal values [20]. Although macrolides have a predominant gastroduodenal site-of-action, they may also induce diarrhea by similar MMC-related mechanisms in the small bowel, and are fully reversible after stopping the drug [21].

Laxatives are drugs used to treat different types of constipation, and may cause diarrhea through a number of mechanisms according to pharmacologic type. Osmotic agents extract through osmosis fluid into the intestinal lumen to soften stools an accelerate colon transit time, examples are non-absorbable carbohydrates (e.g., lactulose), polyethylene glycol, as well as citrate, sodium or phosphate-based products. Stimulant agents induce high-amplitude propagated contractions (HAPC) and alter intestinal and colonic absorption as well as secretion mechanisms, examples include the anthraquinones senna and cascara sagrada, bisacodyl and sodium picosulfate. Newer enterokinetic drugs such as tegaserod and prucalopride are agonists of serotonin 5-HT_4 receptors throughout the GI tract, they also induce increased MMC and HAPC activity and accelerate enteric transit time. Secretagogue agents such as linaclotide, plecanatide, lubiprostone and tenapanor increase intestinal secretion by one of three different mechanisms: activation of intestinal guanylate cyclase C receptors, increasing intraluminal fluid secretion (e.g., linaclotide, plecanatide), type 2 chloride channel activation in the apical membrane of epithelial cells resulting in increased fluid and chloride secretion (e.g., lubiprostone), and inhibition of gastrointestinal sodium-hydrogen exchanger-3 (e.g., tenapanor). All these drugs are used for treating chronic constipation, and IBS with predominant constipation, and diarrhea is the most common side effect. Colchicine is a cytotoxin used to treat acute attacks of gout, and is frequently associated with diarrhea as enhances intestinal water secretion. Misoprostol, a prostaglandin analogue used in the past for drug-associated peptic ulcer disease or in the obstetric practice, is associated frequently with diarrhea induced by an increased smooth-muscle GI activity [22].

5. Dysbiosis

Dysbiosis is a term used to describe any quantitative and/or qualitative imbalance, dysfunction or disturbance of the gut microbiota and microbiome as an indicator of disease or poor health status [23], and may be caused by a number of risk factors, including medications. Drugs and microbiota have a two-way relationship: drugs exert a significant impact on organs and tissues through their effect on gut microbiota, but in the other hand, microbiota metabolic capacity may affect stability, metabolite production, availability, absorption and thus, increase or decrease efficacy and/or toxicity of different medications [24–26]. A number of drugs have been described to alter the composition of the gut microbiota, including antibiotics, proton-pump inhibitors (PPI), nonsteroidal anti-inflammatory drugs (NSAID), opioids, metformin, statins, psychotropics, particularly atypical anti-psychotics, levothyroxine, anticoagulants, antiarrhythmics, and several oncologic medications including chemotherapeutic agents, and targeted therapy [18, 27–33]. A recent study evaluated more than 1000 marketed drugs and found that 24% of them induced significant microbiota composition [30].

5.1 Drugs associated with diarrhea due to dysbiosis

Between 5 and 49% of antibiotic users develop diarrhea during or after treatment. Prevalence is highly variable and can be influenced by reporting country, age, and hospital setting. For instance, antibiotic-associated diarrhea (AAD) represent between 3.2–29% of all causes of diarrhea, with a mean prevalence of 9.6%, in the emergency department this figure raises to 18.6%, and in the intensive care units range from 13.9 to 21.5% [34–36]. Risk factors for AAD are: increasing age, therapy with more than 1 antibiotic, clindamycin use, long-term antibiotic use, and concomitant PPI use. In most cases, withdrawal of antibiotic may stop diarrhea. However, longer use may predispose to enteral and colonic damage, dysbiosis, and increases risk of developing infections by patobionts (microorganisms that usually interact with host in a symbiotic way, but have the potential of acting as pathogens under certain circumstances). Most common microorganisms associated with DAA are *Clostridioides difficile* (formerly known as *Clostridium difficile*), *Klebsiella pneumoniae*, *Clostridium perfringens*, and *Staphylococcus aureus* [37]. Mechanisms associated with DAA can be divided into two main categories: alteration of microbiota/microbiome, and direct effect over intestinal mucosa and motility. Current vision of DAA pathophysiology suggests that antibiotics induce bacterial diversity depletion by at least 30%, with selection of intrinsically resistant micro-organisms, they also may generate gen transfer and de novo mutations conferring resistance to antibiotics. On the other hand, they alter genetic expression, protein activity and cell metabolism, induce under-expression of immunoglobulins, decrease neutrophil and natural killer cell activity, and alter T-cell balance by increasing cytotoxic cells, causing an increased inflammatory tone, that may have a deleterious effect over intestinal permeability [27–29]. *Clostridioides difficile* infection (CDI) is a severe form of DAA with a mixed pathophysiologic model including altered host immune factors, bacterial virulence factors, altered intestinal microbiome and metabolic environment [38]. It has been described a decreased microbial diversity, a direct effect over intestinal permeability, a positive effect on toll-like receptor expression and activation, immune system dysregulation, an altered short-chain fatty acid synthesis, as well as an effect on biliary salts increasing bacterial sporulation/germination capacity [25]. Multiple antibiotics have been linked to ICD, particularly clindamycin, which increase odds ratio almost up to 47 times, but different groups of antibiotics such as amoxicillin/clavulanic acid, aztreonam, cefalosporins, ampicillin, fluoroquinolones, macrolides and even tetracycline may increase risk of ICD [39]. During the last 2 years since the beginning of the SARS-COV-2 pandemics, an increasing incidence of ICD has been reported as widespread antibiotic use and abuse [40–42]. Infection with SARS-COV-2 is associated with two patterns of diarrhea: an early stage, mainly associated to infection itself, apparently caused by direct functional damage of columnar epithelium, and mediated by angiotensin-converting enzyme 2 (ACE-2) receptor interference [40, 42], and a mid to late stage, occurring weeks thereafter, mainly associated with antibiotic use and is related to secondary dysbiosis. A cohort of infected patients that developed diarrhea during the weeks and months following the infection were evaluated, and an AAD prevalence of 16.7% was reported during the follow-up time, with 70% of those developing ICD. In that study, medications associated with increased risk of CDI were amoxicillin (OR 2.2), clarithromycin (OR 3.7), as well as prolonged systemic steroid use (OR 4.4), a drug known for decreasing systemic inflammatory response and immunity [41].

Proton pump inhibitors (PPI) inhibit gastric acid secretion through irreversible blockage of the hydrogen-potassium pump in the parietal cell, and are used for a number of conditions associated with acid exposure such as gastroesophageal reflux disease, peptic-ulcer disease and associated bleeding, and certain types of dyspepsia, and are one of the most common used drugs worldwide [43]. Chronic associated hypochloridria may induce significant changes in microbiota composition throughout the whole gastrointestinal tract. At small intestine long-term PPI use is associated with increasing abundance of *Streptococcaceae*, *Staphylococcaceae*, *Enterobacteriaceae*, *Clostridiaceae*, and decreased abundance of *Bifidobacteriaceae*, and an increased risk for small intestine bacterial overgrowth (SIBO), a condition defined by the presence of more than 10 [5] bacteria per ml of duodenal aspirate and characterized by chronic malabsorptive diarrhea has been reported [31, 44, 45]. In the large bowel, prolonged PPI use also reduces microbial diversity, increasing abundance of *Proteobacteria*, and may also increase risk of CDI (OR 2.3), apparently as a result of a combined pro-inflammatory environment and altered bile-acid homeostasis [45, 46].

A number of different drugs such as atypical anti-psychotics, antidepressants and other mood stabilizers, statins, antiarrhythmics, and anticoagulants are associated with changes in microbiome composition, but its role as a cause of diarrhea is unclear [30, 47, 48]. In several cases, in statins for instance, microbiome changes may be associated with improved outcomes, such as better lipid control [47], in others, as with psychotropics, resulting dysbiosis is associated with anti-commensal activity and drug metabolism alterations, resulting in minor GI symptomatology [30, 48]. Finally, NSAID and immunotherapy are drugs involved in enteropathy by different mechanisms, including dysbiosis, but as mucosal damage is their main pathophysiologic mechanism, are discussed below.

6. Mucosal damage

Drug-associated gastrointestinal damage may affect any part of the GI tract, and small intestine and colon enteropathy accounts for 20–40% of all GI side effects [10]. Mechanisms include direct cytotoxic damage on the intestinal mucosa resulting in several degrees of inflammation, including mucositis, erosions and/or ulcers, hemorrhagic enteritis, alterations in permeability, protein-loss associated enteropathy, and ischemic damage, either caused by long-standing vasoconstriction and/or thrombosis [11]. In some cases, as with chemotherapeutic agents, bone marrow damage and neutropenia may lead to intestinal bacterial translocation, secondary infections with pathogens such as *Pseudomonas* and fungi, resulting in neutropenic enteritis [49]. Another group of inflammatory conditions characterized by microscopic changes only, without endoscopic abnormalities, may affect any part of the GI tract. When small intestine is the affected organ, the condition is called microscopic enteritis, it is manifested usually by chronic diarrhea, anemia and micronutrient deficiencies, and may present with a variety of histological findings with different inflammatory infiltrates –eosinophilic, lymphocytic, or both, collagen deposits, and in some cases, mucosal atrophy. A number of drugs can be associated with this type of microscopic inflammation, affecting small intestine (i.e., angiotensin inhibitors), colon (PPI, selective serotonin release inhibitor antidepressants (SSRI)), or both (aspirin, NSAID) [50, 51].

6.1 Drugs associated with diarrhea due to macroscopic enteral mucosal damage

Non-steroidal anti-inflammatory drugs (NSAID) are prescribed for a variety of pain and inflammation-associated conditions such as rheumatologic and orthopedic disorders, migraine as well as post-surgical states, and exert their effects through cyclooxygenase (COX) inhibition with resultant decrease of prostaglandin synthesis. NSAID are associated both with upper and lower GI symptoms, as well as mucosal injury at any part of the GI tract, and symptoms vary widely from dyspepsia and heartburn to diarrhea, bloating and overt GI bleeding [7, 8, 11, 52–55]. Despite gastroduodenal damage is the most common clinical presentation in most NSAID long-term users, up to 70% may develop different degrees of mucosal breaks, including erosions, ulcerations, mucosal hemorrhage or even stenosis in distal portions of the small intestine such as jejunum or ileum, as determined by studies using video capsule endoscopy [56, 57]. Pathophysiology of NSAID-induced enteropathy is a complex one, and includes different mechanisms such as COX inhibition and topical effect, interactions with bacteria and bile acids, as well as overexpression of pro-inflammatory cytokines. Inhibition of COX-1 is associated with decreased mucosal blood flow, mucus production, and intestinal motility, which are predominant, but not critical factors for damage. Topical effect, a COX-independent action requiring mucosal contact of the drug from the luminal side, is considered the triggering event in most cases [53, 54]. Once NSAID is absorbed into the cell, induces mitochondrial injury by producing vacuolation and swelling, and alters oxidative phosphorylation and electron transport, considered one of the earliest intracellular changes after NSAID administration. As a result, intestinal permeability is increased, allowing luminal factors to disrupt the intestinal barrier function [54]. A second mechanism is associated with interactions between microbiota, bile acids and further activation of innate immunity after being exposed to NSAID. Animal models have shown that germ-free rats treated with NSAID do not develop intestinal ulcers unless bacteria are introduced. NSAID induce an increase in Gram-negative bacterial abundance, *Clostridium* spp. and *Enterobacterococci*. It is well known that Gram-negative bacterial lipopolysaccharides either activate or inhibit toll-like receptors (TLR), leading to inflammatory cascade activation. It has been suggested that antibiotics against Gram-negative bacteria may be effective in reducing NSAID-induced enteral damage [58]. Some bile acids have shown to induce a pro-inflammatory state associated with interleukin-8 (IL-8) and nuclear factor-κβ activation (NF-κβ) activation [54]. Degree of enteral damage varies according to NSAID type and their effect over COX isoforms: non-selective NSAID such as diclofenac, naproxen, meloxicam, or indomethacin inhibits both COX-1 (a constitutive enzyme involved in mucosal integrity), and COX-2 (an isoform primarily inducible related to inflammation), and therefore exert effects through several mechanisms, including topical and systemic effect, as well as dysbiosis. Naproxen have been associated with increased enteral permeability, while indomethacin induces overexpression of the pro-inflammatory tumor necrosis factor-α (TNF-α). NSAID enterohepatic circulation also plays a role in enteral damage, as many are carboxylic acids conjugated in the liver and excreted to bile, cleaved by beta-glucoronidases in the small bowel lumen, and lately reabsorbed. Acetylsalicylic acid (e.g., aspirin), even at low doses, may induce small bowel mucosal breaks after 2 weeks of therapy, mainly due to direct contact damage. On the other part, selective COX-2 inhibitors (ICOX-2) such as celecoxib and etoricoxib have their effect only over the inflammatory isoform, sparing COX-2 and thus, reducing significantly the risk of mucosal damage, unless they are given for prolonged periods of time, after which may have similar risk to that seen with conventional NSAID [7, 11, 53, 54, 58, 59]. Several approaches may diminish the risk of NSAID-induced enteropathy, including withdrawal of drugs, use of selective ICOX-2, or NSAID at the lower therapeutic dose and for short periods of time, or combination with probiotics such as Lactobacillus casei, VSL#3, and S. boulardii, as well as misoprostol, a prostaglandin analog. PPI are not indicated for either prophylaxis nor therapy, and may indeed increase the risk of intestinal injury, apparently associated with changes in microbiota composition [60]. Novel intestinal-sparing NSAID known as co-drugs, consist of two portions: the "NSAID portion" and a gaseous mediator portion (based on nitric oxide or hydrogen sulfide) that exerts mucosal protective effect while sparing therapeutic effect [53]. Further studies are needed to prove their long-term safety in the GI tract.

In addition to NSAID, several drugs may induce small intestine mucosal disease secondary to vasoconstriction and ischemia, including potassium supplements, oral contraceptive pills, and a number of cytotoxic drugs such as methotrexate and chemotherapeutic agents that are associated with different degrees of mucositis [11], and are discussed below.

Among patients receiving oncologic therapy, those treated with cytotoxic drugs, radiotherapy, targeted therapy, and immunotherapy, particularly with the so-called check-point inhibitors have increased risk of developing various degrees of enteropathy and diarrhea. Between 40 and 100% of cancer patients treated with chemotherapeutic agents develop gut toxicity at some point during their treatment, a term called "chemotherapy-induced intestinal mucositis" (CIM). Prevalence and severity depend on drug and dosing regimen, intensity, route of delivery, and patient predisposing conditions. CIM pathophysiology involves mainly mechanisms related to cell growth inhibition, immunological reactions, and dysbiosis [61]. Cytotoxic agents such as methotrexate, doxorubicin, 5-fluorouracil, capecitabin and irinotecan target enteral tissue by interrupting DNA synthesis by direct injury or by generation of reactive oxygen species, leading to release of active signaling factors (i.e., caspases, β-catenin, and NF-κβ), and eventually to mucosal damage and apoptosis, most of which wipe out the intestinal crypt stem cell pool [61, 62]. A five-stage model for CIM has been proposed, that includes: 1) initiation, 2) signal activation and primary damage response, 3) pathway amplification, 4) tissue inflammation (e.g., erosions, ulcerations, apoptosis), and 5) healing. Clinical picture varies widely, and ranges from short periods of diarrhea and abdominal pain, to severe degrees of enterocolitis. When bone marrow-targeted chemotherapeutic agents are also given, increased risk of neutropenic enterocolitis, abdominal sepsis, and even death may occur. Treatment options, beside adjusting dose or even withdrawal of the drug may include antibiotics and probiotics in order to restore normal gut microbiota and reduce pathogenic intestinal bacteria, octreotide to decrease peptide-associated intestinal secretions, antioxidants such as amifostine, a drug that detoxifies reactive metabolites and scavenges free radicals, steroid anti-inflammatory agents to reduce inflammatory response, and possibly incretins and anti-apoptotic agents, most of which are under investigation [11, 61, 62].

Radiation therapy plays an important role as sole curative therapy for 25% of all cancers, and as adjuvant with chemotherapy in many other cases. During radiotherapy of abdominal and/or pelvic tumors, either the small intestine, colon or both are included in the treatment field and may be prone to toxicity. Risk factors for gut damage include those related to therapy itself such as radiation dose, time-dose-fractionation parameters, volume, and concomitant chemotherapy, and patient-related factors such as advanced age, previous abdominal surgeries, as well as vascular and metabolic comorbidities. Radiation enteropathy is classified as early or delayed when occurs prior or after 3 months after treatment. Early symptoms are nausea and abdominal pain, while diarrhea occurs usually after 2 or 3 weeks of treatment onset, and may persist for longer periods of time. Mechanisms of damage are multifactorial and include increased production of reactive oxygen species, mitotic cell death, mucosal atrophy, endothelitis, microvascular sclerosis, as well as fibrosis of the entire bowel wall. As radiation affects predominantly rapidly proliferating intestinal cells, villus epithelium turnover is insufficient to keep normal absorptive mechanisms. Long-term side-effects may include nutrient malabsorption, anemia, stenosis, and in most severe cases, intestinal obstruction. Management is largely symptomatic, with anti-diarrheal agents. As one of the early mechanisms of damage is production of reactive oxygen species, free radical scavengers such as amifostine can be used for reduction of radiotherapy side effects, but it has a narrow therapeutic time window and potential life-threathening side effects. Several candidate mitigator drugs are under investigation [63].

The immune system has an important role in recognizing and eliminating some tumors. Activation of T cells require a signal between T-cell receptors and the major histocompatibility complex along with a stimulatory checkpoint expressed on T cells called CD-28, and the antigen-presenting cells [64]. Tumors may use immune-checkpoint pathways as a mechanism of immune resistance. Two well-known immune-checkpoint receptors are CTLA-4 (CD152), a negative regulator of T-cell-mediated anti-tumor response, and the programmed cell death protein 1 (PD-1 or CD279), expressed on the surface of activated T cells that interacts with programmed death ligand (PD-L1 and L2), leading to T-cell inactivation [64, 65]. The immune check-point inhibitors (ICI) are monoclonal antibodies that block these pathways, including inhibitors of PD-1, PD-L1, and CTLA-4. Immunomodulating therapy, or immunotherapy act to enhance anti-tumor immune responses by blocking negative regulators of immunity, and has revolutionized cancer therapy by improving survival outcomes and is now the standard treatment of different types of cancer, including several metastatic tumors. Currently approved ICI are the anti-PD-1 pembrolizumab and nivolumab, used for treating melanoma and metastatic non-small-cell lung cancer, the anti-CTLA-4 ipilimumab, a fully humanized monoclonal antibody approved for metastatic melanoma, as well as the anti-PDL-L1 atezolizumab and durvalumab, also for non-small cell lung cancer. Ipilimumab, for instance, competitively binds to CTLA-4, blocking tolerance to self-antigens, without blocking CD28 (a stimulatory checkpoint), increasing T-cell proliferation and activation leading to autoimmune damage to a number of organs, including the entire GI tract. In a similar way, anti-PD1/PDL-1 agents such as nivolumab and pembrolizumab increase T-cell response while reducing self-tolerance, and the result is similar to that seen with ipiliumumab [64–67]. This kind of damage behaves similarly to that seen on inflammatory bowel diseases (IBD) such as Crohn's disease and ulcerative colitis, as well as their clinical presentation, with various degrees of enteral and/or colonic damage ranging from erosions and ulcerations to obstruction, and wall necrosis, and presenting as chronic diarrhea, abdominal pain, GI bleeding and progressive anemia [68]. Histologic findings range from combined acute (e.g., neutrophils) and chronic (i.e., lymphocytes and plasma cells) inflammatory infiltrates, eosinophilia, atrophy, granulomatous reaction, crypt abscesses, and bullous pemphigoid, and in most severe cases an increased apoptotic activity within the crypt epithelium may be seen, affecting small intestine, colon or both [69, 70]. Treatment is similar to that given for IBD and may include mesalazine, systemic corticosteroids, and in refractory cases, biologic therapy with infliximab [71, 72].

Another category of oncologic treatment is the called targeted therapy, which acts by identifying and attacking certain types of cancer cells, and by inhibiting oncogenes driving aberrant growth, and may include monoclonal antibodies and small molecule inhibitors. A number of targeted therapies are approved for different types of cancer. Many of them may be associated with different degrees of oral and GI mucositis, particularly cetuximab, erlotinib, gefitinib, lapatinib, sorafenib, and sunitinib, with odds ratio for diarrhea and enteritis ranging from 1.5 to 4.5 [73]. More recently, the HER-2-targeted monoclonal antibody trastuzumab, used for HER-2-overexpressing breast cancer, has been associated with a number of GI manifestations associated to toxicity, including diarrhea, abdominal pain, and ulcerative enterocolitis similar to that seen with ICI. Mechanism underlying GI toxicity remains under investigation, but it seems to be associated with HER-2 receptors in gut epithelial cells [74]. Treatment is empiric, following the same principles as for ICI.

6.2 Drugs associated with diarrhea due to microscopic enteral mucosal damage

A number of drugs are associated with an increased risk of microscopic enteritis and/or colitis, in some cases eosinophilic enteritis, or even may resemble microscopic enteral damage of other diseases, such as celiac disease. Microscopic enteritis encompasses a group of disorders characterized by microscopic mucosal and/or mucosal inflammatory infiltrates by a number of different inflammatory cells, including lymphocytes (i.e., lymphocytic enteritis/colitis), eosinophils (e.g., eosinophilic enteritis/colitis), and lymphocytes along with collagen deposits (i.e., collagenous sprue/collagenous colitis), in absence of significant macroscopic mucosal damage, leading to watery diarrhea [50, 75–77]. In the small bowel, microscopic enteritis may also be associated with mucosal atrophy in some cases, and the clinical picture may be that of malabsorptive diarrhea, with foul-smelling feces, steatorrhea, and anemia [76]. In most cases an autoimmune predisposition has been proposed, but when disease develops during or shortly after a specific drug use, causality for drug-induced disease can be proposed according to a World Health Organization system based on temporal sequence, prior information of the drug, dose–response relationship, exclusion of other etiologies, and re-challenge [78]. Pathophysiology mechanisms are not clear, and may involve activation of the immune system in response to exposure to luminal antigenic factors, including drug-itself, metabolites, bile-acids, or may be associated with changes in microbiota linked to long-term drug use, such as in PPI.

A number of drugs have been linked to microscopic colitis, including aspirin, NSAID, PPI, SSRI, particularly sertraline, clozapine, ticlopidine, flavonoids and acarbose [51]. A recent case–control study found a significant increased risk for microscopic colitis with current use of NSAID, PPI, and SSRI with adjusted odd ratios of 1.86, 3.37 and 2.03 respectively. Current PPI use was associated also with increased risk of both lymphocytic (OR 2.06) and collagenous colitis (OR 5.3), whereas current NSAID use was associated with increased risk of collagenous colitis (OR 2.32), and current SSRI use increased risk of lymphocytic colitis (OR 2.28). Long-term PPI and/or NSAID use had the highest odds ratio (4.6 and 4.8 respectively) for developing microscopic colitis [79]. As previously mentioned, NSAID may affect any part of the GI tract, by a number of different pathophysiologic mechanisms. In the small intestine NSAID-associated damage ranges from microscopic enteritis to severe mucosal affection with erosions and/or ulcers. Histologic manifestations of NSAID may resemble those of celiac disease, with villous blunting and intraepithelial lymphocytosis, and can be found in any part of the small intestine [80].

Eosinophilic enteritis and colitis are included in the group of eosinophilic gastrointestinal disorders, and are characterized by a high eosinophilic infiltrate in the gut wall, without evidence of other causes. Pathophysiology involves a combination of genetic predisposition, dysbiosis, and a triggering factor, usually an allergen, that may include drugs, followed by recruitment and activation of eosinophils to sites of inflammation regulated by pro-inflammatory cytokines [81]. Drugs such as clozapine, naproxen, carbamazepine, and rifampicin have been associated with increased eosinophilic infiltrate in the distal ileum and colon [77]. More recently the anti-CTLA-4 check-point inhibitor ipilimumab and the anti-PD1 nivolumab have been link to eosinophilic enteritis [70]. Other immunosuppressant drugs such as mycophenolate mofetil, a drug used to prevent acute allograft rejection may affect both small bowel and colon, causing an eosinophilic-associated damage, with features similar to those of acute graft-versus-host disease [82].

Angiotensin II receptor inhibitors (AT-II RI) are one of the most common drugs for treating high blood pressure, with a generally safe side-effect profile. In 2012 a case series of 22 patients developing chronic diarrhea and weight loss while taking olmesartan was published. None had positive celiac serology, and a combination of villous atrophy and variable degrees of inflammation including collagen deposits was observed in small intestine biopsies, with clinical and histologic recovery after discontinuation of the drug [83]. More recently, other AT-II RI have been also associated with different degrees of enteropathy. A systematic review included 248 cases, most of which were associated with olmesartan (94%), however telmisartan, irbesartan, valsartan, losartan and eprosartan also were reported to be associated with various degrees of enteropathy. Interestingly, despite negative serology in most cases, 71% had a positive HLA-DQ2 or DQ-8, haplotypes associated with celiac disease [84].

7. Conclusion

Drugs are a common cause of chronic diarrhea and enteropathy by a number of mechanisms including intrinsic mode of action, malabsorption, dysbiosis, increased GI motility, alterations in water and electrolyte absorption and secretion mechanisms, autoimmune macroscopic or microscopic damage, and cytotoxic effect. Site of damage may include either part of the small intestine, colon, or both, and can be manifested by malabsorptive, inflammatory or watery diarrhea. In most cases diarrhea subsides after drug withdrawal, but in some cases a number of inflammatory conditions requiring other forms of therapy may be needed.

Author details

Octavio Gómez-Escudero
Hospital Angeles Puebla, Puebla, Mexico

*Address all correspondence to: octavio_gomezmd@yahoo.com.mx

References

[1] Aranda-Michel J, Gianella RA. Acute diarrhea: A practical review. The American Journal of Medicine. 1999;**106**:670-676

[2] Fine KD, Schiller LR. AGA technical review on the evaluation and management of chronic diarrhea. Gastroenterology. 1999;**116**:1464-1486

[3] Lacy BE, Mearin F, Chang L, et al. Bowel disorders. Gastroenterology. 2016;**150**:1393-1407

[4] Schiller LR, Pardi DS, Sellin JH. Chronic diarrhea: Diagnosis and management. Clinical Gastroenterology and Hepatology. 2017;**15**:182-193

[5] Camilleri M, Sellin JH, Barrett KE. Pathophysiology, evaluation, and management of chronic watery diarrhea. Gastroenterology. 2017;**152**:515-532

[6] Gomez-Escudero O, Remes-Troche JM. Approach to the adult patient with chronic diarrhea: A literature review. Revista de Gastroenterología de México. 2021;**86**:387-402

[7] Hamdeh S, Micic D, Hanauer S. Review article: Drug-induced small bowel injury. Alimentary Pharmacology & Therapeutics. 2021;**54**:1370-1388

[8] Chassany O, Michaux A, Bergmann JF. Drug-induced diarrhea. Drug Safety. 2000;**22**:53-72

[9] Murray JA, Rubio-Tapia A. Diarrhoea due to small bowel diseases. Best Practice & Research. Clinical Gastroenterology. 2012;**26**:581-600

[10] Kiela PR, Guishan FK. Physiology of intestinal absorption and secretion. Best Practice & Research. Clinical Gastroenterology. 2016;**30**:145-159

[11] Zeino Z, Sisson G, Bjarnason I. Adverse effects of drugs on small intestine and colon. Best Practice & Research. Clinical Gastroenterology. 2010;**24**:133-141

[12] Clissold SP, Edwards C. Acarbose, a preliminary review of its pharmacodynamic and pharmacokinetic properties and therapeutic potential. Drugs. 1988;**35**:214-243

[13] Moelands SVL, Lucassen PLBJ, Akkermans RP, et al. Alpha-glucosidase inhibitors for prevention or delay of type 2 diabetes mellitus and its associated complications in people at increased risk of developing type 2 diabetes mellitus. Cochrane Database of Systematic Reviews. 2018;**12**:CD005061

[14] Henness S, Perry CM. Orlistat. Drugs. 2006;**66**:1625-1656

[15] Filippatos TD, Derdemezis CS, Gazi IF, et al. Orlistat associated adverse events and drug interactions -a critical review. Drug Safety. 2008;**31**:53-65

[16] Bryson A, de la Motte S, Dunk C. Reduction of dietary fat absorption by the novel gastrointestinal lipase inhibitor cetilistat in healthy volunteers. British Journal of Clinical Pharmacology. 2009;**67**:309-315

[17] Rena G, Grahame Hardie D, Pearson ER. The mechanisms of action of metformin. Diabetologia. 2017;**60**:1577-1585

[18] McCreight LJ, Bailey CJ, Pearson ER. Metformin and the gastrointestinal tract. Diabetologia. 2016;**59**:426-435

[19] Foss MT, Clement KD. Metformin as a cause of late-onset chronic diarrhea. Pharmacotherapy. 2001;**21**:1422-1424

[20] Sanger GJ, Wang Y, Hobson A, Broad J. Motilin: Towards a new understanding of the gastrointestinal neuropharmacology and therapeutic use of motilin receptor agonists. British Journal of Pharmacology. 2013;**170**:1323-1332

[21] Otterson MF, Sarna SK. Gastrointestinal motor effects of erythromycin. The American Journal of Physiology. 1990;**259**:355-363

[22] Bharucha AE, Lacy BE. Mechanisms, evaluation, and management of chronic constipation. Gastroenterology. 2020;**158**:1232-1249

[23] Wei S, Bahl MI, Baunwall SMD, et al. Determining gut microbial dysbiosis: A review of applied indexes for assessment of intestinal microbiota imbalances. Applied and Environmental Microbiology. 2021;**87**:e00395-e00321

[24] Cani PD, Delzenne NM. The gut microbiome as therapeutic target. Pharmacology & Therapeutics. 2011;**130**:202-212

[25] Sousa T, Paterson R, Moore V, et al. The gastrointestinal microbiota as a site for the biotransformation of drugs. International Journal of Pharmaceutics. 2008;**363**:1-25

[26] Gimenez-Batista JA, Martínez L, Moya-Pérez A, Laparra JM. Phramacological efficacy/toxicity of drugs: A comprehensive update about the dynamic interplay of microbes. Journal of Pharmaceutical Sciences. 2018;**107**:778-784

[27] Francino MP. Antibiotics and the human gut microbiome: Dysbiosis and accumulation of resistances. Frontiers in Microbiology. 2016;**6**:1543

[28] Beaugerie L, Petit JC. The gut microflora and the pathogenesis of gastrointestinal disease: Antibiotic-associated diarrhea. Best Practice & Research. Clinical Gastroenterology. 2004;**18**:337-352

[29] Li X et al. Microbiota and diarrhea: An updated review. Frontiers in Cellular and Infection Microbiology. 2021;**11**:625210

[30] Maier L, Pruteanu M, Kuhn M, et al. Extensive impact of non-antibiotic drugs on human gut bacteria. Nature. 2018;**555**:623-628

[31] Bruno G, Zaccari P, Rocco G, et al. Proton pump inhibitors and dysbiosis: Current knowledge and aspects to be clarified. World Journal of Gastroenterology. 2019;**25**:2706-2719

[32] Wang X, Tang Q, Hou H, et al. Gut microbiota in NSAID enteropathy: New insights from inside. Frontiers in Cellular and Infection Microbiology. 2021;**11**:679396

[33] Gaucher L, Adda L, Séjourné A, et al. Associations between dysbiosis-inducing drugs, overall survival and tumor response in patients treated with immune checkpoint inhibitors. Therapeutic Advances in Medical Oncology. 2021;**13**:1-23

[34] Elseviers MM, Van Camp Y, Nayaert S, et al. Prevalence and management of antibiotic associated diarrhea in general hospitals. BMC Infectious Diseases. 2015;**15**:129

[35] Haran JP, Wu G, Bucci V, et al. Antibiotic-associated diarrhea in emergency department observation unit patients. Epidemiology and Infection. 2016;**144**:2176-2183

[36] Zhou H, Xu Q, Liu Y, Guo LT. Risk factors, and morbidity associated with antibiotic-associated diarrhea in

intensive care unit patients receiving antibiotic monotherapy. World Journal of Clinical Cases. 2020;**8**:1908-1915

[37] Polage CR, Solnick JV, Cohen SH. Nosocomial diarrhea: Evaluation and treatment of causes other than Clostridium difficile. Clinical Infectious Diseases. 2012;**55**:982-989

[38] Monaghan TM. New perspectives in Clostridium difficile disease pathogenesis. Infectious Disease Clinics of North America. 2015;**29**:1-11

[39] Teng C, Reveles KR, Obodozie-Ofoegbu OO, Frei CR. Clostridium difficile infection risk with important antibiotic classes: An analysis of the FDA adverse events reporting system. International Journal of Medical Sciences. 2019;**16**:630-635

[40] Sandhu A, Tillotson G, Polistico J, et al. Clostridioides difficile in COVID-19 patients, Detroit, Michigan. Emerging Infectious Diseases. 2020;**26**:2274-2274

[41] Maslennikov R, Svistunov A, Ivashkin V, et al. Early viral versus late antibiotic-associated diarrhea in novel coronavirus infection. Medicine. 2021;**100**:41

[42] Cao TT, Zhang GQ, Pellegrini E, et al. COVID-19 and its effects on the digestive system. World Journal of Gastroenterology. 2021;**27**:3502-3515

[43] Spechler SJ. Proton pump inhibitors, what the internist needs to know. Medical Clinics of North America. 2019;**103**:1-14

[44] Fujimori S. What are the effects of proton pump inhibitors on the small intestine? World Journal of Gastroenterology. 2015;**21**:6817-6819

[45] Bavishi C, Dupont HL. Systematic review: The use of proton pump inhibitors and increased susceptibility to enteric infection. Alimentary Pharmacology & Therapeutics. 2011;**34**:1269-1281

[46] Janarthanan S, Ditah I, Adler DG, Ehrinpreis MN. Clostridium difficile-associated diarrhea and proton pump inhibitor therapy: A meta-analysis. The American Journal of Gastroenterology. 2012;**107**:1001-1010

[47] Dias AM, Cordeiro G, Estevinho MM, et al. Gut bacterial microbiome composition and statin intake – A systematic review. Pharmacology Research & Perspectives. 31 May 2020:e00601. DOI: 10.1002/prp2.601

[48] Cussotto S, Clarke G, Dinan TG, Cryan JF. Psychotropics and the microbiome. A chamber of secrets. Psychopharmacology. 2019;**236**:1411-1432

[49] Wade DS, Nava HR, Douglass HO Jr. Neutropenic enterocolitis, clinical diagnosis and treatment. Cancer. 1992;**1**:17-23

[50] Rostami K, Aldulaimi D, Holmes G, et al. Microscopic enteritis: Bucharest consensus. World Journal of Gastroenterology. 2015;**21**:2593-2604

[51] Lucendo AJ. Drug exposure and the risk of microscopic colitis: A critical update. Drugs. 2017;**17**:79-89

[52] Bjanarson I, Haylla RJ, Macpherson AJ, et al. Side effects of nonsteroidal anti-inflammatory drugs on the small and large intestine. Gastroenterology. 1993;**104**:1832-1847

[53] Wallace JL. Mechanisms, prevention and clinical implications of nonsteroidal anti-inflammatory drug-enteropathy. World Journal of Gastroenterology. 2013;**19**:1861-1876

[54] Watanabe T, Fujiwara Y, Chan FKL. Current knowledge on non-steroidal anti-inflammatory drug-induced small-bowel damage: A comprehensive review. Journal of Gastroenterology. 2020;**55**:481-495

[55] Tai FWD, McAlindon ME. Non-steroidal anti-inflammatory drugs and the gastrointestinal tract. Clinical Medicine. 2021;**21**:131-134

[56] Gay G, Delvaux M, Frederic M. Capsule endoscopy in non-steroidal anti-inflammatory drugs-enteropathy and miscellaneous, rare intestinal diseases. World Journal of Gastroenterology. 2008;**14**:5237-5244

[57] Fujimori S, Gudis K, Takahashi Y, et al. Distribution of small intestinal mucosa injuries as a result of NSAID administration. European Journal of Clinical Investigation. 2010;**40**:504-510

[58] Rekatsina M, Paladini A, Cifone MG, et al. Influence of microbiota on NSAID enteropathy: A systematic review of current knowledge and the role of probiotics. Advances in Therapy. 2020;**37**:1933-1945

[59] Smecuol E, Bai JC, Sugai E, et al. Acute gastrointestinal permeability responses to different non-steroidal anti-inflammatory drugs. Gut. 2001;**49**:650-655

[60] Wallace JL, Syer S, Denou E, et al. Proton pump inhibitors exacerbate NSAID-induced small intestinal injury by inducing dysbiosis. Gastroenterology. 2011;**141**:1314-1322

[61] Dahlgren D, Sjöblom M, Hellström PM, Lennemäs H. Chemotherapeutics-induced intestinal mucositis: Pathophysiology and potential treatment strategies. Frontiers in Pharmacology. 2021;**12**:681417

[62] Peterson DE, Bensadoun RJ, Roila F. Management of oral and gastrointestinal mucositis: ESMO clinical practice guidelines. Annals of Oncology. 2011;**22**(6):vi78-vi84

[63] Hauer-Jensen M, Denham JW, Andreyev HJN. Radiation enteropathy – Pathogenesis, treatment, and prevention. Nature Reviews. Gastroenterology & Hepatology. 2014;**11**:470-479

[64] Som A, Mandaliya R, Alsaadi D, et al. Immune check-point inhibitor-induced colitis: A comprehensive review. World Journal of Clinical Cases. 2019;**7**:405-418

[65] Bellaguarda E, Hanauer S. Checkpoint inhibitor-induced colitis. The American Journal of Gastroenterology. 2020;**115**:202-210

[66] Samaan MA, Pavlidis P, Papa S, et al. Gastrointestinal toxicity of immune checkpoint inhibitors: From mechanisms to management. Nature Review Gastroenterol & Hepatol 2018;**15**: 222-234. DOI: 10.1038/nrgastro.2018.14

[67] Rajha E, Chaftari P, Kamal M, et al. Gastrointestinal adverse events associated with immune checkpoint inhibitor therapy. Gastroenterology Report. 2020;**8**:25-30

[68] Iranzo I, Huguet JM, Suárez P, et al. Endoscopic evaluation of immunotherapy-induced gastrointestinal toxicity. World Journal of Gastrointestinal Endoscopy. 2018;**10**:392-399

[69] Ibraheim H, Perucha E, Powell N. Pathology of immune-mediated tissue lesions following treatment with immune checkpoint inhibitors. Rheumatology (Oxford). 2019;**58**(S7):vii17-vii28

[70] Yang J, Lagana SM, Saenger YM, Carvajal RD. Dual

checkpoint inhibitor-associated eosinophilic enteritis. Journal for Immunotherapy of Cancer. 2019;7:310

[71] Weber JS, Postow M, Lao CD, Schadendorf D. Management of adverse events following treatment with anti-programmed death-1 agents. The Oncologist. 2016;**21**:1-11

[72] Iyoda T, Kurita N, Takada A, et al. Resolution of infliximab-refractory nivolumab-induced acute severe enterocolitis after cyclosporine treatment in a patient with non-small cell lung cancer. American Journal of Case Reports. 2018;**19**:360-364

[73] Elting LS, Chang YC, Parelkar P, et al. Risk of oral and gastrointestinal mucosal injury among patients receiving selected targeted agents: A meta-analysis. Support Care Cancer. 2013;**21**:3243-3254

[74] Al-Dasooqi N, Bowen JM, Gibson RJ, et al. Trastuzumab induces gastrointestinal side effects in HER2-overexpressing breast cancer patients. Investigational New Drugs. 2009;**27**:173-178

[75] Pardi D. Diagnosis and management of microscopic colitis. The American Journal of Gastroenterology. 2017;**112**:78-85

[76] Jansson-Knodell CL, Hujoel IA, Rubio-Tapia A, Murray JA. Not all that flattens villi is celiac disease: A review of enteroathies. Mayo Clinic Proceedings. 2018;**93**:509-517

[77] Impellizzeri G, Marasco G, Eusebi LH, et al. Eosinophilic colitis: A clinical review. Digestive and Liver Disease. 2019

[78] World Health Organization UMC. The use of the WHO-UMC system for standardized case panel causality assessment. Available from: http://who-umc.org/graphics/24734.pdf

[79] Verhaegh BP et al. High risk of drug-induced microscopic colitis with concomitant use of NSAIDs and proton pump inhibitors. Alimentary Pharmacology & Therapeutics. 2016;**43**:1004-1013

[80] Owen DR, Owen DA. Celiac disease and other causes of duodenitis. Archives of Pathology & Laboratory Medicine. 2018;**142**:35-43

[81] Collins MH, Capocelli K, Yang GY. Eosinophilic gastrointestinal disorders pathology. Frontiers in Medicine. 2018;**4**:261

[82] Parfitt JR, Jayakumar S, Driman DK. Mycophenolate mofetil related gastrointestinal mucosal injury: Variable injury pattern including graft-versus-host disease-like changes. The American Journal of Surgical Pathology. 2008;**32**:1367-1372

[83] Rubio-Tapia A et al. Severe sprue-like enteropathy associated with olmesartan. Mayo Clinic Proceedings. 2012;**87**:732

[84] Kamal A, Fain C, Park A, et al. Angiotensin II receptor blockers and gastrointestinal adverse effects of resembling sprue-like enteropathy: A systematic review. Gastroenterology Report. 2019;7:162-167

Chapter 6

Diagnostic Approaches of Dysfunctional Anorectum and Pelvic Floor Disorders

Nikolaos Andromanakos, Dimitrios Filippou and Alkiviadis Kostakis

Abstract

Various causes of neuromuscular disorders of the pelvic floor muscles may affect the functional integrity of the pelvic floor and anorectum leading to the different pathological conditions such as anorectal incontinence, urinary incontinence and constipation of obstructed defecation, sexual dysfunction, and perineal pain syndromes. Diagnosis of the dysfunctional anorectum and pelvic floor disorders is an integrated approach that includes a thorough history, a careful physical examination, and selected specialized tests as well as the exclusion of organic disease (anorectal or endopelvic) which complement the patient's evaluation contributing to objective and accurate diagnosis of their pathological cause leading to the optimal treatment.

Keywords: anorectal incontinence, constipation, dyssynergic pelvic floor, levator ani syndrome, myofascial syndrome, pelvic outlet obstruction, perineal pain

1. Introduction

Variety causes of neuromuscular disorders of the pelvic floor muscles may affect the functional integrity of the pelvic floor and anorectum leading to the different pathological conditions such as anorectal incontinence, urinary incontinence and constipation of obstructed defecation, sexual dysfunction, and perineal pain syndromes.

Anorectal incontinence is considered a severe condition that influences the patient's life causing mainly unsafety as well anxiety and fear to social contact. The exact incidence of anorectal incontinence is unknown but in a few epidemiological studies it has been reported 2.2–8.3% in the population. It is more frequent in women and particularly in the elderly. However, some studies reported an incidence >50% [1–3].

Constipation can significantly affect the quality of patient' life and its diagnosis may be done at every age but usually in the elderly and in women. The incidence of chronic constipation has been calculated in epidemiological studies 2–27% [4, 5]. The Rome III diagnostic criteria have been helped to constipation definition (**Table 1**) [6]. However, constipation is assumed a subjective symptom of varied pathological conditions (**Table 2**) [7]. Furthermore, constipation can be distinguished in normal constipation, slow transit constipation, and constipation of pelvic outlet obstruction or obstructed defecation [8]. Constipated patients with obstructed defecation usually have a normal colonic transit time, but delayed transit in the rectosigmoid part [9]. Some of these patients are presented with a megarectum, large rectocele, enterocele, rectal prolapse, or perineal descent, while others maintain a spasm of the pelvic floor muscles leading to difficult evacuation [10].

Perineal pain syndromes are characterized by chronic perineal pain (anorectum and perineum) without anorectal or endopelvic organic disease [11]. These syndromes constitute an idiopathic multifactorial complex interaction between neurological, musculoskeletal, and endocrine systems that is more influenced by psychological and behavioral factors [12]. The lack of understanding of the etiology of perineal pain is evident in its many names (chronic perineal, pain chronic idiopathic anal pain,

Symptom onset at least 6 months before diagnosis
Presence of symptoms in the last 3 months
Diagnosis includes two or more symptoms at least 25% of defecations
• Straining
• Lumpy or hard stools
• Feeling of incomplete evacuation
• Feeling or anorectal obstruction or blockage
• Manual maneuvers to facilitate evacuation

Table 1.
Rome III criteria to diagnosis of chronic constipation.

Anorectum and pelvic floor
• Neoplasms, polyps
• Megarectum
• Anal stenosis
• Mucosal rectal prolapse
• Internal rectal prolapse
• Complete rectal prolapse
• Solitary rectal ulcer
• Rectocele
• Enterocele
• Descending perineum syndrome
• Hirschsprung's disease
• Anismus
• Dyssynergic pelvic floor
• Hereditary internal anal sphincter myopathy

Table 2.
Causes of constipation of obstructed defecation.

anorectal neuralgia, levator syndrome, spastic pelvic floor syndrome, spastic levator syndrome, and spastic piriformis) which endeavor to describe the problem [13]. McGivney and Cleveland published an article in 1993 entitled "Levator syndrome and its treatment" [14]. However, the knowledge of the anatomy and physiology of the pelvic floor is of the sine qua non to understand the pathophysiology of chronic perineal pain syndromes [15].

In this review study we present diagnostic approaches of the dysfunctional anorectum and pelvic floor disorders which are accompanied by elements of their etiology and pathophysiology contributing to objective patients' assessment and to accurate diagnosis of their pathological cause that lead to the appropriate treatment selection.

2. Dysfunctional anorectum and pelvic floor disorders

2.1 Idiopathic anorectal incontinence

Neurogenic anorectal incontinence is considered idiopathic, especially in women, because it may be due to damage of the nerves innervating the pelvic floor muscles. Causes of idiopathic anorectal incontinence are usually associated with difficult childbirth, constipation with chronic straining at stool, rectal prolapse, descending perineum syndrome, and advanced age. Pathophysiology of idiopathic anorectal incontinence is attributed to traction of the pudendal nerve or compression of the sacral nerves by the pelvic floor that descends or to pressure by the fetal head. Evidence that idiopathic incontinence relates to denervation injury of the pelvic floor seems clearly in manometry, electromyography, and pudendal nerve latency studies. These studies show that idiopathic incontinence is characterized by weakness of the pelvic floor and anal canal musculature [16].

2.2 Constipation of functional obstructed defecation

Constipation of functional obstructed defecation may be associated with anismus or dyssynergic pelvic floor, megarectum, Hirschsprung's disease, and descending perineum syndrome. Anismus is characterized as a pelvic floor dysfunction. The puborectalis muscle and external anal sphincter fail to relax or paradoxically contract during straining to defecate leading to a difficult or impossible defecation. Dyssynergic pelvic floor is characterized by incoordination of the abdominal, rectoanal, and pelvic floor muscles leading to difficult or incomplete evacuation. The pathophysiological mechanism of persistent constipation is the failure of the anorectal angle to open, of the perineum to descend and of the anal canal to shorten as a result of sustained contraction of the puborectalis muscle [17]. Megarectum is a rare condition that is differentiated from Hirschsprung's disease with rectal biopsies. Patients with megarectum often suffer from constipation (fecal impaction). In these cases there may be an impaired rectal sensation and high distensibility. In addition, impaired rectal sensation and ignoring or resisting the physiological urge to defecate lead to accumulation of more stools in the rectum, which are difficult and painful to expel [18]. Hirschsprung's disease is another type of pelvic outlet obstruction which is characterized by absence of rectoanal inhibitory reflex. Aganglionosis leads to loss of internal anal sphincter relaxation when the rectum is distended [19, 20]. Descending perineum syndrome is characterized by a persistent and intractable difficulty to defecate. Abnormal perineal descent during straining to defecate is probably secondary to injury to pudendal and sacral nerves from trauma, childbirth, or chronic straining at defecation [21, 22].

2.3 Perineal pain syndromes

Perineal pain syndromes are characterized by anorectal and perineal pain without anorectal or endopelvic organic disease which should be excluded. The most common perineal pain syndromes are levator ani syndrome, proctalgia fugax, and myofascial syndrome which are characterized by a chronic or recurrent anorectal and perineal pain. Etiology of these syndromes is usually idiopathic. However, they may relate to pelvic injury (fall, accident, and childbirth), surgical procedures (prostatectomy, hysterectomy, low anterior resection, spinal column, and anal fistulae), prolonged sitting in a car or train or hard surface, excessive physical activity, psychological stress, anxiety, and sexual abuse. Pathophysiology of levator ani syndrome is similar to that of dyssynergic defecation (incoordination between anorectum and pelvic floor muscles during defecation). The failure of relaxation of levator ani (puborectalis) or the external anal sphincter muscles or paradoxical contraction of them during straining to defecate was called spastic pelvic floor syndrome. Pathophysiology of proctalgia fugax has been associated with spasm of pelvic floor, abnormal contractions of internal anal sphincter, and hypertrophy of internal anal sphincter (inherited myopathy). Pathophysiology of myofascial syndrome relates to "trigger points" which are connected with the disturbance of the nerve endings and an abnormal contractile mechanism at many dysfunctional endplates. These endplates constitute the sites of active trigger points [23].

2.4 Evaluating patients with dysfunctional anorectum and pelvic floor disorders

In the diagnostic approach of dysfunctional anorectum and pelvic floor disorders (idiopathic incontinence, constipation of functional obstructed defecation, and perineal pain syndromes) that contribute to the history, a careful physical examination, specialized investigations, and the exclusion of anorectal or endopelvic organic disease should be carried out. In incontinent patients, the history may elicit leaking of enteric content (gases, fluid stool, or formed stool) and record the frequency, duration, severity, and timing of incontinence episodes. The incontinence may be true or false (over flow diarrhea), passive (neurogenic incontinence) or uncontrolled (diarrhea, trauma of anal sphincter, or puborectalis). However, a past medical history (obstetric, anorectal surgeries, constipation with straining at stool, rectal prolapse, low back pain, sciatica, and medications) should carefully be assessed. On physical examination should be looked for signs of incontinence. Perineal inspection (at rest and strain) may show perianal soiling, patulous anus, scars, prolapsing hemorrhoids, perineal descent, or rectal prolapse. The absence of anocutaneous reflex indicates pudendal neuropathy. Digital rectal examination may reveal tumors or impacted stool and at the same time allows the internal and external sphincter function evaluation (at rest and squeeze) as well as anorectal ring of the puborectalis assessment by palpation. Rectosigmoidoscopy should always be carried out to exclude neoplasms, proctitis, internal rectal prolapse, or a solitary rectal ulcer. At the end of the patient's interview should be determined the degree of incontinence (mild, moderate, and severe) and then some specialized tests should be recommended, if necessary. This can be done using a proposed incontinence scoring system (e.g., Wexner, Pescatori, and Altomare) [24–26]. Thus, clinical evaluation is complemented by anorectal physiology tests (anorectal manometry, anal endosonography (AES), pudendal nerve terminal motor latency (PNTML), defecography, electromyography (EMG), and MRI) which provide objective patients' assessment and accurate diagnosis of the incontinence cause contributing to the appropriate treatment. However, in clinical practice, anorectal manometry, AES, and PNTML have been shown to be the most useful tests in diagnosis and after-treatment follow up [27, 28]. Anorectal manometry is the first investigation for anorectal physiology which may assess the anal sphincters function (at rest and squeeze), rectal sensation, and rectoanal reflex. In incontinence, anal canal pressures (at rest and squeeze) are low with or without impaired rectal sensation. Rectal sensation disorder may be managed by biofeedback [29]. AES is another examination in the diagnosis of anorectal incontinence, providing information about the anal sphincters integrity [30]. PNTML assesses the pudendal nerve function. Prolongation of PNTML is considered the diagnostic evidence of idiopathic incontinence [31]. Defecography is a useful test which may show anatomical and functional abnormalities of the anorectum and pelvic floor contributing to the anorectal angle assessment that is obtuse in idiopathic incontinence patients [32]. However, the recently used dynamic MRI of the pelvic floor in defecatory disorders may be a more efficient alternative to traditional defecography [33]. Furthermore, recent studies suggest that the defecography can also be replaced by perineal ultrasound [34]. EMG may detect functional anal sphincter abnormalities in incontinent patients with normal AES [35]. In constipated patients, the history may derive valuable information concerning the characteristics of patient's symptoms, the duration, and severity (difficult, painful, incomplete, or impossible defecation) but also the stool frequency, stool consistency, and stool size. A past medical history, obstetric, surgery, neurological, psychological, or medicines should be recorded. However, a recent history of severe constipation or overflow diarrhea in elderly should be carefully investigated to exclude an organic pathology (neoplasm) or impacted stool. Physical examination includes examination of the abdomen, perineum, and anorectum. Abdomen examination should exclude an intra-abdominal mass or tenderness. Perineal inspection may reveal a patulous anus, soiling, scars, prolapsing hemorrhoids, fistulas, or fissure. Digital examination may detect stool (fecal impaction), stricture, or neoplasm and at the same time should be done an anal sphincter function assessment (at rest, squeeze, and straining). If not observed pelvic floor dysfunction (pelvic outlet obstruction or dyssynergia), unusual perineum bulging or rectal prolapse may be noticed. Furthermore, an anterior rectocele or enterocele should be sought. Physical examination should always be followed by rectosigmoidoscopy which can identify anorectal and colonic pathologies (stricture, neoplasm, internal rectal prolapse, megarectum, inflammatory bowel disease, or solitary rectal ulcer). However, diagnostic approach of constipated patient is completed by selected specialized investigations which can diagnose and differentiate with accuracy and objectivity the constipation causes of obstructed defecation leading to optimal treatment. Specialized tests include colonic transit time test, anorectal manometry, defecography, balloon expulsion test, and EMG. In addition, new specialized techniques as high-resolution anorectal manometry, dynamic MRI, and dynamic perineal ultrasound have been used and proved useful in the diagnostic attempt of the dysfunctional disorders cause of the anorectum, pelvic floor, and colon [36–39]. Colonic transit time is estimated by an abdominal X-ray 5 days after using radiopaque markers. Retention of the markers in the rectosigmoid colon suggests a dyssynergic pelvic floor and pelvic outlet obstruction [40].

Anorectal manometry (at rest and straining) may show motor dysfunction of the anorectum (impaired anal relaxation-anal resting pressure unchanged) or (paradoxical anal contraction-anal resting pressure increases), or both [41, 42] and sensory dysfunction of anorectum (impaired rectal sensation and high distensibility-threshold for first sensation and for call to defecate elevated) in constipation of obstructed defecation [43, 44]. Rectoanal inhibitory reflex is usually present except in Hirschsprung's disease that is absent [45]. However, the new technique of high-resolution anorectal manometry seems to have more advantages compared with conventional manometry (easier use, more accurate values of the anorectal pressures, complete anorectal imaging, and automatic analysis of the recording results with color morphology) allowing a most comprehensive diagnostic approach of the dysfunctional anorectum and pelvic floor disorders as idiopathic incontinence, dyssynergic pelvic floor, and Hirschsprung's disease [46–48]. Defecography, in patients with functional obstructed defecation, may show acute anorectal angle as an inability of puborectalis muscle relaxation or a spastic pelvic floor [49, 50]. However, recently, dynamic MRI of the pelvic floor and dynamic perineal ultrasound can be considered an alternative to traditional defecography [51]. In balloon expulsion test, patients with obstructed defecation are unable to expel the balloon [52]. EMG can recognize a dysfunctional puborectalis or/and external anal sphincter, in cases with obstructed defecation (anismus or dyssynergia) during straining, recording to increased their pathological activity [53, 54]. In patients with perineal pain syndromes, in the diagnostic approach of patients with chronic perineal pain an important place occupy the thorough history, careful physical examination, and selected specialized tests. Perineal pain syndromes are clinically distinguished by the duration of painful episodes, frequently, and characteristics. However, perineal pain of dysfunctional pelvic floor syndromes should be distinguished by pelvic pain. Pelvic pain usually relates to pathological conditions such as gynecological or urological diseases, infection, irritable bowel disease, and neurological disorders. All these pathological conditions may affect the perineal muscles (pelvic floor, anal, and urethral sphincters) and sometimes may pretend dysfunctional syndromes with perineal pain, as the levator ani syndrome. So, the history may give useful information about the characteristics of pain, the location, duration, frequency, provocative factors, and factors of worsening the pain. Furthermore, the past medical history (medicines, pelvic injury, surgical procedures, excessive physical activity, psychological distress, anxiety, psychical trauma, sexual abuse, and psychical disease) should be recorded. Physical examination includes inspection and palpation of the perineum. Digital rectal and vaginal examination is significant in the assessment of the anorectum and levator ani muscle (puborectalis). The diagnosis of dysfunctional pelvic floor syndromes is based on characteristics symptoms, digital examination findings of levator ani palpation (tenderness, contraction, or sensitive trigger points), pathological tests as electromyography and exclusion of the anorectal or endopelvic organic disease with perineal pain. Nevertheless, the diagnosis of these syndromes may be difficult because they constitute overlapping functional entities. The differential diagnosis of chronic perineal pain includes neoplasms of anorectum, anal fissure, anorectal abscess, thrombosed external hemorrhoids, proctitis, cystitis, endometriosis, internal rectal prolapse, descending perineum syndrome, solitary rectal ulcer, leukemia, and neurological disorders spinal column or spinal cord [23].

In conclusion, diagnostic approaches of dysfunctional anorectum and pelvic floor disorders include the history, a careful physical examination and selected specialized tests as well as the exclusion of the anorectal or endopelvic organic disease that contribute to objective and accurate diagnosis of their pathological cause leading to the optimum treatment.

Conflict of interest

The authors declare that they have no competing interests.

Author details

Nikolaos Andromanakos[1*], Dimitrios Filippou[2] and Alkiviadis Kostakis[3]

1 Department of General Surgery, Lefkos Stavros Athens Hospital, Athens, Greece

2 Department of Anatomy and Surgical Anatomy, Athens, Greece

3 Biomedical Research Foundation of Athens Academy, Athens, Greece

*Address all correspondence to: n.andromanakos@gmail.com

References

[1] Leung FW, Rao SS. Fecal incontinence in the elderly. Gastroenterology Clinics of North America. 2009;**38**:503-511

[2] Whitehead WE, Borrud L, Goode PS, Meikle S, Mueller ER, Tuteja A, et al. Fecal incontinence in US adults: Epidemiology and risk factors. Gastroenterology. 2009;**137**:512-517

[3] Nelson R, Norton N, Cauttey E, Furner S. Community-based prevalence of anal incontinence. JAMA. 1995; **224**:559-561

[4] Dennison C, Prasad M, Lloyd A, Bhattcharyya SK, Dhawan R, Coyne K. The health related quality of life and economic burden of constipation. PharmacoEconomics. 2005;**23**:461-476

[5] Sanchez MI, Bercik P. Epidemiology of berden of chronic constipation. Canadian Journal of Gastroenterology. 2011;**25**(Suppl. B):11B-15B

[6] Drossman DA. The functional gastrointestinal disorders and the Rome III process. Gastroenterology. 2006;**130**:1377-1390

[7] Seltzer R. Evaluation and diagnosis of constipation. Gastroenterology Nursing. 2012;**35**:343-348

[8] Foxx-Orenstein AE, McNally MA, Odunsi ST. Update on constipation: One treatment does not fit all. Cleveland Clinic Journal of Medicine. 2008;**7**:813-823

[9] Wald A. Severe constipation. Clinical Gastroenterology and Hepatology. 2005;**3**:432-435

[10] Toglia MR. Pathophysiology of anorectal dysfunction. Obstetrics and Gynecology Clinics of North America. 1998;**25**:771-781

[11] Ger GC, Wexner SD, Jorge JM, Lee E, Amaranath LA, Heymen SM, et al. Evaluation and treatment of chronic intractable rectal pain—A frustrating endeavor. Diseases of the Colon and Rectum. 1993;**36**:139-145

[12] Gunter J. Chronic pelvic pain: An integrated approach to diagnosis and treatment. Obstetrical & Gynecological Survey. 2003;**58**:615-623

[13] Neil ME, Swash M. Chronic perineal pain: An unsolved problem. Journal of the Royal Society of Medicine. 1982;**75**:96-101

[14] McGivney JO, Cleveland BR. The levator syndrome and its treatment. Southern Medical Journal. 1965;**58**:505-510

[15] Finamore P, Goldstain H, Whitmore K. Pelvic floor muscle dysfunction: A review. Journal of Pelvic Medicine and Surgery. 2008;**14**:417-422

[16] Andromanakos N, Filippou D, Pinis ST, Kostakis A. Anorectal incontinence: A challenge in diagnostic and therapeutic approach. European Journal of Gastroenterology & Hepatology. 2013;**25**:1247-1256

[17] Andromanakos N, Pinis ST, Kostakis A. Chronic severe constipation: Current pathophysiological aspects, new diagnostic approaches and therapeutic options. European Journal of Gastroenterology & Hepatology. 2015;**27**:204-214

[18] Araghizadeh F. Fecal impaction. Clinics in Colon and Rectal Surgery. 2005;**18**:116-119

[19] Aaronson I, Nixon HH. A clinical evaluation of anorectal pressure studies in the diagnosis of Hirschsprung's disease. Gut. 1972;**13**:138-146

[20] Moore BG, Singaram C, Eckhoff DE, Gaumnitz EA, Starling JR. Immunohistochemical evaluation of ultrashort-segment Hirschsprung's disease. Report three cases. Diseases of the Colon and Rectum. 1996;**39**:817-822

[21] Snooks DJ, Setchell M, Swash M. Injury to innervation of pelvic floor sphincter musculature in childbirth. Lancet. 1984;**2**:546-550

[22] Kiff ES, Barnes PB, Henry MM. Prolongation of pudendal nerve latency and increased single fibre density in patients with chronic defecation straining and perineal descent. The British Journal of Surgery. 1983;**70**:681

[23] Andromanakos N, Kouraklis G, Kostakis A. Chronic perineal pain: Current pathophysiological aspects, diagnostic approaches and treatment. European Journal of Gastroenterology & Hepatology. 2011;**23**:2-7

[24] Jorge JM, Wexner SD. Etiology and management of fecal incontinence. Diseases of the Colon and Rectum. 1993;**36**:77-79

[25] Pescatori M, Anastasio G, Bottini C, et al. New grading and scoring for anal incontinence. Evaluation of 335 patients. Diseases of the Colon and Rectum. 1992;**35**:482-487

[26] Altomare DF, Di Lena M, Giuratrabocchetta S, Giannini I, Falagario M, Zbar AP, et al. The three axial perineal evaluation (TAPE) score: A new scoring system for comprehensive evaluation of pelvic floor function. Colorectal Disease. 2014;**16**:459-468

[27] Rao SS. Diagnosis and management of fecal incontinence. The American Journal of Gastroenterology. 2004;**99**:1585-1604

[28] Seong MK, Jung SI, Kim TW, Joh HK. Comparative analysis of summary scoring system in measuring fecal incontinence. Journal of the Korean Surgical Society. 2011;**80**:326-331

[29] Pehl C, Seidl H, Scalercio N, Gundling F, Schmidt T, Schepp W, et al. Accuracy of anorectal manometry in patients with fecal incontinence. Digestion. 2012;**86**:78-85

[30] Pinsk I, Brown J, Phang PT. Assessment of sonography quality of anal muscles in patients with faecal incontinence. Colorectal Disease. 2009;**11**:933-940

[31] Ricciardi R, Mellgren AF, Madoff RD, Baxter NN, Karulf RE, Parker SC. The utility of pudendal nerve terminal motor latencies in idiopathic incontinence. Diseases of the Colon and Rectum. 2006;**49**:852-857

[32] Jones HJ, Swift RI, Blake H. A prospective audit of the usefulness of evaluating proctography. Annals of the Royal College of Surgeons of England. 1988;**80**:40-45

[33] Fletcher JG, Busse RF, Riederer ST, Hough D, Gluecker T, Harper CM, et al. Magnetic resonance imaging of anatomic and dynamic defects of the pelvic floor in defecatory disorders. The American Journal of Gastroenterology. 2003;**93**:399-411

[34] Zufferey G, Pemeger T, Robert-Yap J, Skala K, Roche B. Accuracy of measurement of puborectal contraction by perineal ultrasound in patients with faecal incontinence. Colorectal Disease. 2011;**13**:e234-e237

[35] Tjandra JJ, Milson JW, Schroeder T, Facio VW. Endoluminal ultrasound is preferable to electromyography in mapping anal sphincter defects. Diseases of the Colon and Rectum. 1993;**96**:689-692

[36] Jamshed N, Lee ZE, Olden KW. Diagnostic approach of chronic constipation in adults. American Family Physician. 2011;**84**:299-306

[37] Bove A, Pucciani F, Bellini M, Battaglia E, Bocchini R, Altomate DF, et al. Concensus statement AIGO/SICCR: Diagnosis and treatment of chronic constipation and obstructed defecation (part I: diagnosis). World Journal of Gastroenterology. 2012;**14**:1555-1564

[38] Lacy BE, Levenick JM, Crowell M. Chronic constipation: New diagnostic and treatment approaches. Therapeutic Advances in Gastroenterology. 2012;**5**:233-247

[39] Tack J, Muller-Lissner S, Stanghellini V, Boeckxstaens G, Kamm MA, Simren M, et al. Diagnosis and treatment of chronic constipation—A European perspective. Neurogastro enterology and Motility. 2011;**23**:697-710

[40] Metcaff AM, Phillips SF, Zinsmeister AR, MacCarty RL, Beart RW, Wolff GB. Simplified assessment of segmental colonic transit. Gastroenterology. 1987;**92**:40-47

[41] Park UK, Choi SK, Piccirillo MF, Verzaro R, Wexner SD. Patters of anismus and the relation to biofeedback therapy. Diseases of the Colon and Rectum. 1996;**39**:768-773

[42] Perera LD, Ananthakrishnan AN, Guilday C, Remshak K, Zadvomova Y, Naik AS, et al. Dyssynergic defecation: A treatable cause of persistent symptoms when inflammatory bowel disease is inremission. Digestive Diseases and Sciences. 2013;**58**:3600-3605

[43] Gosselink MJ, Schouten MR. Rectal sensory perception in females with obstructed defecation. Diseases of the Colon and Rectum. 2001;**44**:1337-1344

[44] Rasmussen OO, Sorensen M, Tetzschner T, Christiansen J. Dynamic anal manometry in the assessment of patients with obstructed defecation. Diseases of the Colon and Rectum. 1993;**36**:901-907

[45] Chen F, Winston JH, Frankel WL. Hirschsprung's disease in a young adult: Report of a case and review of the literature. Annals of Diagnostic Pathology. 2006;**10**:347-351

[46] Jones MP, Post J, Crowell MD. High-resolution manometry in the evaluation of anorectal disorders: A simultaneous comparison with water-perfused manometry. The American Journal of Gastroenterology. 2007;**102**:850-855

[47] Xu C, Zhao R, Conklin JL, Yang X, Zhang Y, Zhang X, et al. Three dimensional high-resolution anorectal manometry in the diagnosis of paradoxical puborectalis syndrome compared with healthy adults: Prospective study in 79 cases. European Journal of Gastroenterology & Hepatology. 2014;**26**:621-629

[48] Wu JF, Lu CH, Yang CH, Tsai IJ. Diagnostic role of anal sphincter relaxation integral in high-resolution anorectal manometry for Hirschsprung disease in infants. The Journal of Pediatrics. 2018;**194**:136-141

[49] Somorowska E, Henrichen S, Christiansen J, Hegedus V. Video-defecography compared with measurement of anorectal angle and perineum descent. Acta Radiologica. 1987;**28**:559-562

[50] Canechan A, Anderson EM, Upponi S, Planner AC, Slater A, Moore N, et al. Imaging of obstructed defecation. Clinical Radiology. 2008;**63**:18-26

[51] Vitton V, Vignally P, Barthet M, Cohen V, Durieux O, Bouvier M, et al. Dynamic anal endosonography and MRI defecography in diagnosis of pelvic floor disorders: Comparison with conventional defecography. Diseases of the Colon and Rectum. 2011;**54**:1398-1404

[52] Deck DE. Simplified balloon expulsion test. Diseases of the Colon and Rectum. 1992;**35**:597-598

[53] Stalberg E, Kouyoumdjian J, Sanders D. Reference values in concentric needle electrode studies. Clinical Neurophysiology. 2013;**124**:1255-1256

[54] Harverson AL, Orkin BA. Which physiologic tests are useful in patients with constipation? Diseases of the Colon and Rectum. 1998;**41**:735-739

Chapter 7

Perspective Chapter: Surgical Management of Symptomatic Rectocele

Esther María Cano Pecharromán, A. Teresa Calderón Duque, Juan Carlos Santiago Peña and Tomás Balsa Marín

Abstract

Rectocele is defined as a herniation of the anterior rectal wall through the posterior vaginal wall into the vaginal lumen caused by rectovaginal septum weakness. This entity is more common in postmenopausal female patients. Approximately one-third of adult women affected with pelvic organ prolapse have a significant impact on their quality of life and emotional well-being. Up to more than 90% of woman can be asymptomatic. In symptomatic cases, constipation, defecatory disorders such as obstructed syndrome (ODS) or incontinence, vaginal mass, and pelvic discomfort are the main complaints. Surgical treatment is indicated after failure of conservative management. Talking about ODS, nearly 20% of the patients need surgery. Surgical options can be classified as abdominal (being laparoscopic colposacropexy the technique of choice) or perineal approach. In the latter group, the alternatives are transanal (TA), transperineal (TP), and transvaginal (TV) approaches with or without prosthetic material or grafts. Native-tissue transvaginal approach should be preferentially performed as it has shown better results. Nowadays, there is no consensus on what the gold-standard technique is given the lack of strong evidence.

Keywords: symptomatic rectocele, rectocele treatment, surgical approach, transvaginal approach, comparison

1. Introduction

Rectocele is defined as a herniation of the anterior rectal wall through the posterior vagina wall into its lumen, caused by weakness of the rectovaginal septum. It is more common in postmenopausal women, and pelvic organ prolapse can occur in more than 50% of parous women [1–4]. Usually secondary to multiple vaginal deliveries that may cause pelvic floor injuries, or damages in muscles such as the levator ani or at the rectovaginal septum, even or the pudendal nerve.

In many cases, more than 90%, it is asymptomatic [1]. The symptoms caused by the rectocele may be related to defecatory disorders, constipation, vaginal mass or bulge and pelvic discomfort, and even in some occasions mild fecal incontinence with

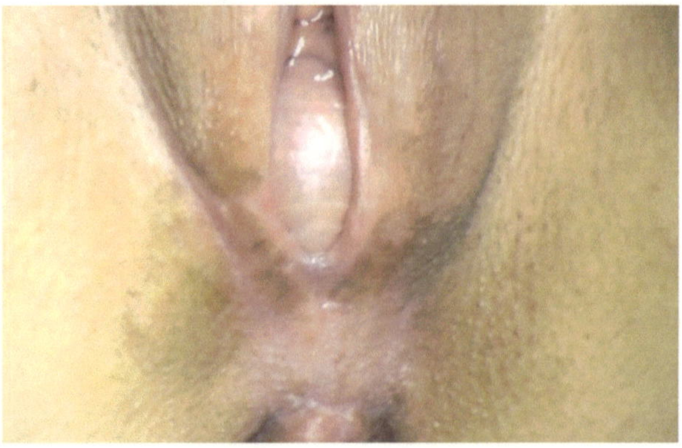

Figure 1.
Physical examination of rectocele. The superior part of the picture shows the anterior part of the patient, and the inferior part of the picture shows the posterior part of the patient (anal area).

soiling symptoms. It should be considered as a cause of the well-known Obstructed Defecation Syndrome (ODS) [4]. Thus, in a large percentage of women with rectocele, from 30 to 70% [5], they present symptoms such as difficulty in rectal emptying, excessive straining to defecation, or the need for vaginal digitation to complete defecation.

Despite this relationship, it should be remembered that ODS is a multifactorial entity, and many etiologies have already been related to it. For example, pelvic floor dyssynergia, rectal prolapse, intussusception, and pelvic floor prolapse are some of

Transvaginal (TV)	Posterior colporrhaphy +/– levatorplasty	Without mesh (longitudinal/transverse/purse-string closure)
		With mesh biologic/Synthetic (resorbable or non-absorbable)
	Site-specific repair	
	Iliococcygeus fascia suspension	
Transperineal (TP)	Manual suture	
	Sperr	
Transanal (TA)	Hand sewing	Sarles.
		Sullivan
		Khubchandani
	Stapled suture	Starr-transtar
		TRREMS
		Khubchandani's procedure
Abdominal (laparoscopic/robotic/open)	Colpoperineopexy	
	Iliococcygeus fascia suspension	
Mixed	Sacral colpopexy or iliococcygeus fascia suspension + colporrhaphy	

Table 1.
Classification scheme of surgical techniques for rectocele repair.

them. Thus, despite optimal surgical correction of the rectocele, part of the initial symptoms such as sexual dysfunction, dyspareunia, or constipation could persist (**Figure 1** and **Table 1**).

The diagnosis of rectocele is initially clinical, after a correct anamnesis and physical examination of the entire pelvic floor, ruling out other "celes" or associated pathologies. In addition, we must assess possible gynecological alterations, the integrity of the rectovaginal septum and anatomical defects or the tone of the anal sphincter and identify neurological lesions. An anoscopy can help to rule out a possible associated intussusception. The severity of symptoms should be evaluated with standardized scores such as the "Obstructed Defecation syndrome" score or the "Pelvic Organ Prolapse Scoring system" POP-SS. This should include associated symptoms such as urinary incontinence or fecal incontinence with validated scales, e.g., "Wexner Score" (Cleveland Clinic Incontinence Score). Additionally, the impact on the quality of life should be considered and measured through the numerous existing questionnaires.

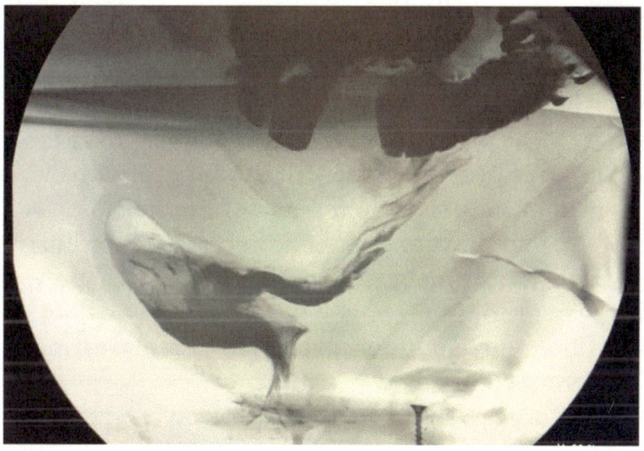

Figure 2.
Videodefecography.

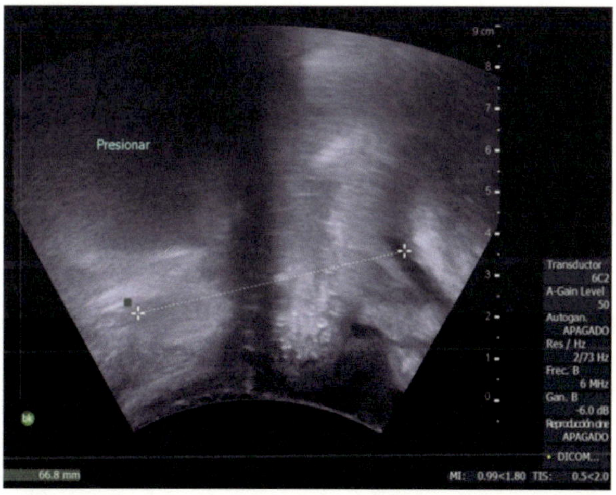

Figure 3.
Perineal ultrasound. It is usually performed in lithotomy position, with an empty rectum and with an optimums Valsalva maneuver of 6 seconds [6].

Regarding the complementary examination, it may be useful to perform a defecography, currently considered the gold-standard test to diagnose pelvic organ prolapse or a dynamic pelvic resonance imaging (MRI). The latter have a high sensitivity of around 100% for the diagnosis of rectocele and a specificity of 57%. Rectocele is currently recognized as a classic indication for this test. Considering that the rectocele can be physiological when performing Valsalva maneuver, it is considered physiological in the imaging tests if it is asymptomatic and smaller than 2.5 cm (**Figures 2** and **3**).

Another technique that can be performed in case of incontinence associated or alterations of the anal sphincter suspected is the endoanal of perineal ultrasound [3, 4].

2. Conservative treatment

Initial management is conservative and symptomatic. Different non-surgical options can be offered. Those conservative treatments are taken into consideration for cases with a mild degree of prolapse [7, 8]. The treatment choice depends on the profile of the patient (conservative treatment is considered too for frail patients), on how symptomatic is the prolapse, the severity of it, or the preferences of the patient.

The interventions can be physical or lifestyle. The first group is based on the hypothesis that an improvement of the structural support por pelvic organs will occur due to the improvement of the pelvic floor muscle function.

That means exercise to train strength, endurance, and coordination of the pelvic floor contractions, as the Cochrane review about conservative prevention and management of pelvic organ prolapse in women named as "pelvic floor muscle training" [8]. This way pelvic floor rehabilitation can be a successful treatment for rectocele or even recto-rectal intussusceptions.

In cases of small rectocele, there may be a regression in a percentage of cases, so observation should be considered while starting conservative treatment, not being the case in large rectoceles, which do not usually return. Talking about ODS, around 20% [2] of the cases need surgical treatment, taking into account that the cause of it can be the reflection of many other pathologies apart from rectocele, such as anismus, rectal hypo sensation, anxiety, or depression.

Hygienic-dietetic measures should be taken in case of constipation, such as increased water intake, a diet rich in fiber, even oral laxatives, which are the most used alternatives. Foods that increase the viscosity may be avoided.

Another alternative reported as effected for several authors is hydrocolontherapy or lavage. It consists in irrigation through a tube into the anorectum. We have to take into account that the abuse of enemas can cause microtrauma and anorectal fibrosis secondarily [2].

Biofeedback or pelvic floor training helps to increase the quality of the pelvic floor muscles and therefore the support of the pelvic organs, it is also a treatment with hardly any adverse effects [8], and it is more indicated in cases of anismus and rectal hypo sensation, as well as botulinum toxin A treatment [2]. The use of electrostimulation is used in pudendal neuropathy and rectal hyposensation. Physiological counseling should be offered and can be helpful in several patients with depression or anxiety. Psycho-echo-biofeedback has been recently proposed as a procedure that is successful in half of the cases [2].

The use of the pessary can be recommended, usually in patients older than 70 years, serving as a support, occupying the space in lieu of the rectocele. It can improve symptoms of pressure, feeling of occupation and mass, even urinary ones in up to 50% of cases. There are different types of pessaries that can be adapted to the patient situation as their sexual life, active or not.

3. Surgical indication

SDO can have many causes as already explained, one of them is the pudendal nerve injury and secondary pelvic floor denervation. One of the factors that can contribute to the development of fecal or urinary incontinence is denervation of the muscles such as puborectalis, pubococcygeus, and pelvic fascia [8, 9]. Some studies link decreased pudendal nerve function and incontinence in women [10]. In that sense, delivery-related pelvic floor trauma [9] can result in pelvic muscle or fascia trauma and pudendal nerve injury. There are electromyography and pudendal nerve conduction studies after childbirth showing denervation [11].

Other factors such as chronic straining at stool are related to pudendal nerve injury. This affection is being studied as it can have an association with genuine stress incontinence. Women with low urinary tract dysfunction have more chance of suffering from SDO symptoms, which makes think of benign joint hypermobility syndrome or other connective tissue disorders as an important factor [12].

Considered all the possible causes, surgical treatment in patients with obstructive defecation symptoms is indicated after having completed a conservative management, and this has not achieved control of the symptoms and, after it has been provided that there is an anatomical basis that justifies them.

In the specific case of patients with ODS, the origin could be a functional disorder, and we must demonstrate an anatomical cause through imaging that justifies the intervention. The surgical indications for a rectocele are normally a size longer than 3 cm [3], or a significant retention of the barium contrast within it, during defecography associated with important symptoms that affect quality of life, such as the need for frequent digitation to achieve defecation [13]. Prior to the indication for surgery, it is essential to inform the patient and determine the expectations that the patient has of the surgical treatment [14].

4. Surgical treatment techniques and approaches

Once surgery is indicated, the technique will be decided based on the characteristics of the rectocele and the patient, as well as their preferences. The approach could be abdominal or extra-abdominal (perineal) approach and within the latter group: transanal, transperineal, or transvaginal, with variations in each of them [1]. We could summarize them schematically as follows:

The main objective of the surgery is focused on correcting the anatomical defect, and secondarily improving the symptoms of obstructive defecation [15]. There is a wide variety of techniques described in the literature, including those referred to above, which can be associated with the performance of flaps or placement of prosthetic material such as meshes, either biological or synthetic [4].

There is not enough evidence available in most studies to suggest that one surgical technique or approach is better than another, and therefore, despite the data presented, it is important that each surgeon performs the technique with which you are more familiar and have more experience.

Existing data support the recommendation to consider posterior colporrhaphy of native tissue by transvaginal approach as first surgical option in cases of female patients with rectocele and obstructive defecation symptoms and with surgical indication. This improves anatomical defects and obstructive defecation symptoms. Although, evidence shows that the anatomical defect of the prolapse may persist over time, and symptomatic improvement may decrease in long-term follow-up. Despite this, more studies will be needed to recommend a surgical technique as the "gold standard."

Therefore, overall, the advice given to patients may be given under the premise that most of the techniques described have an improvement from both the anatomical and symptomatic point of view in terms of ODS symptoms, without the existence of a single type of surgery that stands out above the others [15].

5. Abdominal approach

In the main abdominal approach (Colpoperineopexy), an opening of the pelvic peritoneum is performed, and a non-absorbable mesh is placed in the rectovaginal septum, attaching the top of the vagina on the sacral promontory. In the case of also performing the pexy of the rectum on its anterior or posterior face, it will be called colporectosacropexy (**Figure 4**). It can be performed using a minimally invasive approach such as laparoscopic or robotic, which is why this technique has been more popular in recent years.

This technique shows improvement in ODS (> 70%) with low morbidity and low recurrence rates (7.5 and 14.2% in 3 and 10 years, respectively) [3]. Although there is an anatomical improvement after surgery, there are studies that report that, however, this improvement is not reflected in defecation symptoms and may even worsen [15]. Thus, this technique is indicated mainly in patients with complex rectocele or invagination or associated rectal prolapse and symptoms of ODS.

In very few cases of ODS, no damage to the posterior wall is associated, which is corrected with vaginal apical pexy. In these cases, laparoscopic ventral rectopexy can be performed, indicated in patients with enterocele or ODS secondary to rectal intussusception [4].

When rectal prolapse is associated, techniques such as Frykman-Goldberg technique can be used. This technique, described in 1969, combines rectopexy and resection of the redundant sigma with anastomosis [16].

In this technique, a rectal dissection must be performed low on the posterior vaginal wall for a subsequent pexy "to the periosteum of the sacral promontory" once the rectum is freed and mobilized, as described in the reference [16]. After the pexy, the redundant sigmoid colon resection and the anastomosis are performed. It is therefore, a technique recommended in cases in which there is a constipation due to a redundant sigma existence or due to the rectum angulation. It is also used in cases in which the surgeon avoids placing meshes taking into account the associated risk as in pregnancies.

In the absence of an ideal mesh for intra-abdominal placement, we prefer the perineal approach in cases of celes in the posterior compartment and the abdominal approach with direct pexy to the sacrum in case of several compartments involvement, avoiding the use of mesh as much as possible.

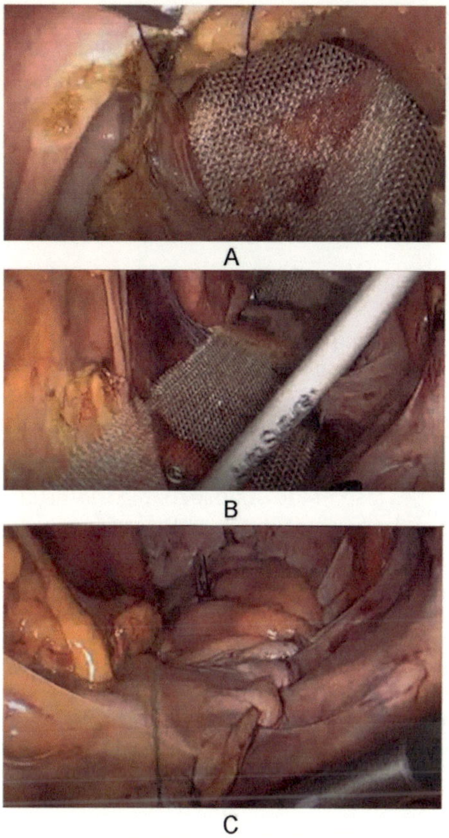

Figure 4.
Rectocolposacropexy: (A), (B). Laparoscopic mesh placement and fixation with PDO stitches and tackers to sacral promontory. (C) Peritoneum closure.

Frykman-Goldberg surgery can be performed by open, laparoscopic, or robotic approach [17]. However, in this chapter we focus on extra-abdominal techniques.

6. Extra-abdominal approach

6.1 Transperineal approach

The transperineal extra-abdominal technique begins with the infiltration of saline serum and adrenaline at the level of the rectocele, to facilitate its dissection. After that, transverse perineal incision is performed, and the plane between the external anal sphincter and the posterior vaginal wall is dissected with either blunt or sharp dissection [13].

Once the apex of the vagina is reached and the exposure of the rectocele and the levator muscle is completed, the upper limit of the rectocele is identified as the point at which it differs from the longitudinal muscle of the lower rectus wall. A plication of the rectocele is performed in the midline from the most apical point downwards, successive plications can be performed. The plication can be vertical or horizontal, presenting better results the horizontal according to Waleed et al. [18]. Levatorplasty may or may not be associated. Finally, the cutaneous plane is closed after the reconstruction of the rectovaginal septum.

6.2 Transanal approach

Within the transanal approach, there are classic techniques performed by and sewing such as transanal rectoceleplasty, and others more innovative in which mechanical sutures are used.

6.2.1 Hand sewing

Transanal rectoceleplasty [19] is classically performed in the jackknife position and with prior retrograde preparation with a cleansing enema and an anal retractor. After infiltration of saline with epinephrine, a transverse incision is made in the dentate line, and a muco-muscular flap with a broad base is made about 7–10 cm proximally. After careful revision of hemostasis, successive plications are performed, first longitudinally and later transversely with absorbable material (plyglicolic acid) sutures. After resecting the excess part of the flap, it is completed with the closure of the flap with simple stitches also made of absorbable material.

Other transanal rectoceleplasties have specific variations in their technique, such as those described below: In the Sarles technique, an opening of the mucosa is performed over the rectocele and subsequently a transverse plication of the rectal muscle layer is performed.

In the Sullivan technique, a horizontal plication is performed with several sutures.

The Khubchandani technique is a mixed technique in which a stapler suture is performed on the posterior rectal wall and subsequently a U-shaped flap and after that transverse and vertical plicatures on the anterior wall [5].

Regarding results, transanal approach achieves an anatomical improvement of the defect and the symptoms of obstructive defecation. Infection is more common in this technique as a complication [15]. In addition, it can also compromise the function of the anal sphincter [19], which in this case may cause de novo incontinence.

6.2.2 Mechanical suture (stapled)

Continuing on the topic of transanal approach, we will discuss the technique of transanal rectal resection with stapler (stapled transanal rectal resection STARR) [15].

The STARR technique involves double stapling with a circular stapler and an anal dilator and a purse-string suture. It is performed through a transanal approach in order to achieve a circumferential resection of the entire thickness of the anterior and posterior rectal wall. There are modifications in which the resection of the rectal wall is performed with an endostapler, or with the CONTOUR®TRANSTARTM semi-circular stapler, a technique called TRANSTAR, which can facilitate the resection of the entire thickness of the rectal wall and is considered a safe and effective treatment for ODS (STARR TRANSTAR) associated with rectal wall intussusception and/or rectocele in the hands of experienced surgeons [20].

The STARR technique has positive impact in anatomical and obstructive defecation symptoms. The most frequent adverse effects and complications are urgency fecal incontinence, in up to 40%, that usually improves with time and resolves in about 3 months, minor bleeding, and postoperative pain [15]. Other important but infrequent complications are rectal diverticulum, rectovaginal fistula, rectal obliteration, rectal wall hematoma, or perforation. These complications appear to be reduced by using a parachute suture instead of a purse-string suture [20]. The existence of various ways or tricks in this type of approach is a sign of the real need for standardization of the technique.

The TRREMS (transanal repair of rectocele and rectal mucosectomy with one circular stapler) [21] performs the section with a single circumferential stapler, and it is suggested as a safe, economic, and effective procedure for the treatment of rectocele associated with mucosal prolapse.

Within the techniques performed with a stapler, there is a transperineal variation that consists of the mechanical stapling of the rectocele with a GIA, after dissecting the rectovaginal septum, adding a reinforcing PLP mesh at this level. This technique is called SPERR (Stapled Perineal Rectocele Resection).

6.3 Transvaginal approach

For a century, posterior transvaginal **colporrhaphy** and its modifications have been the usual transvaginal approach with optimal anatomical results.

In lithotomy position, and after infiltration of the vaginal wall with saline and adrenaline to facilitate dissection and reduce bleeding, a transverse incision is made at the level of the mucocutaneous junction (vaginal introitus) in the posterior vaginal wall. Annex 1 shows the main steps of this technique shown in a real case.

Dissection of the rectovaginal septum is continued, combining blunt and sharp dissection, until reaching the proximal end of the rectocele and laterally until exposing the puborectal muscles [4, 13].

After completing the dissection, the rectovaginal septum and the rectal wall are plicated in a longitudinal direction with simple stitches, using a non-absorbable polypropylene suture (prolene®), long-term absorbable monofilament (PDO), or absorbable polyglycolic acid braided suture. 2/0.

In the case presented as an example in Annex 1, it was combined with the previous performance of purse-string plications with vicryl® suture at the point of maximum protrusion of the rectocele, given the large size of this specific case. In case of an associated enterocele, the sac is opened after dissection and subsequently closed, hence repositioning the Douglas sac.

Perineorrhaphy with horizontal sutures and levatorplasty may be associated or omitted. It is important to check both the consistency of the rectovaginal septum and the correct size of the vagina post plication by rectal and vaginal examination, some authors propose at least two fingers in diameter.

Finally, the excess tissue of the vaginal mucosa flap is excised, which is done in the exposed case after marking the section level using indocyanine green. However, the use of this technology is not imperative. Finally, the closure of the vaginal plasty is completed with simple absorbable sutures. It is not necessary to place drains in the closure.

Regarding the results [15] of posterior colporrhaphy with native tissue, the literature shows that an improvement in anatomical and obstructive defecation symptoms is achieved after this technique. Side effects or complications have a low incidence, being dyspareunia the most common.

After the exposition of the main techniques, the existence of **Site-Specific Repair** [15] should be explained. This technique also improves anatomical defects and most obstructive defecation symptoms, but its results in terms of constipation are unclear. The most common side effects are dyspareunia and also tenesmus.

Specifically in the transvaginal approach, with the use of non-absorbable synthetic meshes, post-surgical complications have been described. There is a wide variety in terms of the severity of these complications, from pain, infection, bleeding, granulomas, urinary tract infection, dyspareunia, and even extrusion of the mesh or formation of fistulas or visceral lesions such as rectal, bladder, or vaginal perforation (1–4%). In the long term, up to 30% of patients may present mesh contraction with pain and dyspareunia [22].

FDA (Food and Drug Administration) has made a safety communication concerning about this topic, making a recommendation for the use of mesh in the transvaginal approach only "after weighing the risks and benefits of surgery with mesh versus all surgical and non-surgical alternatives" [23]. So, it should be used only in complex cases after failures of other surgeries and providing information about the possibility of all possible complications.

7. Techniques comparison

Even though there is no clear conclusion that one surgical technique is superior to the rest, there are numerous studies that compare existing techniques to address the need for consensus on what the recommendation should be.

The inferiority of the site-specific repair technique is clear, since posterior colporrhaphy has shown better anatomical results and in terms of symptoms in comparison, so this technique should not be used as a first-choice technique.

Regarding the transperineal approach, it has been recommended in combination with sphincteroplasty or levatorplasty for the treatment of symptomatic rectocele. These procedures have resulted in improved evacuation and continence in 75% of patients. Regarding the transvaginal repair, it provides better results of anatomical repair of the rectocele and fewer recurrences. Both techniques are associated with significant postoperative dyspareunia rates [15].

In a 2020 randomized study [2, 13] comparing the transperineal approach with the transvaginal approach for the treatment of anterior rectocele, it was determined that the transvaginal repair of the rectocele achieved an improvement in constipation and quality of life related to function sexual compared with the transperineal approach. There were no significant changes in dyspareunia. From the point of view of intraoperative time, postoperative complications, and recurrence, no significant differences were found.

Posterior transvaginal colporrhaphy with native tissue compared with the transanal approach presents better anatomical results in vaginal examination but not in defecography, with improvement in terms of constipation and incomplete evacuation without changes in terms of digitation needs, with similar rates of complications [15].

It is important to consider certain anatomical aspects such as in the case of the transvaginal approach, there is no direct interference with the anal canal, so that the involvement of the anal sphincter is very unlikely, compared with the transanal approach. Therefore, this technique can be given priority in patients with previous damage or pathologies in the anal sphincter.

Certain authors attach importance to the caliber of the vagina in the face of post-surgical dyspareunia. This is not a trivial complication, and it occurs in more than

33% of sexually active women after performing different rectocele repair techniques. Other comparisons show a significant improvement in the sexual satisfaction of patients after a transvaginal approach but not after a trans perineal approach, possibly due to the change in the anatomy of the vagina or "rejuvenation" that occurs in the first technique and not in the second [15].

When it comes to the use of native tissue versus biological flaps, no anatomical improvements of the posterior compartment or symptomatic improvements of ODS have been observed, and there are no differences in terms of complications. There are also no better anatomical or symptomatic results with the use of synthetic meshes. Their use presents complications such as dyspareunia or erosions and even mesh extrusion in the case of a transvaginal approach.

8. Conclusion

There is not a superior technique that can be recommended as the only "gold standard." For this reason, the surgical treatment of the rectocele must be individualized in each case according to the needs of the patient and surgeon's experience.

A transvaginal approach with posterior colporrhaphy and native tissue is recommended in cases of women with ODS who require surgical treatment, reporting the rate of possible post-surgical dyspareunia.

In cases with multicompartmental prolapse or with a very high rectocele, an abdominal approach is more suitable (**Figure 5**).

Non-absorbable mesh should not be used in the vaginal approach due to potential adverse effects.

An improvement in the results with the use of biological materials has not been demonstrated; however, their use increases the surgical costs.

Site-specific repair has a higher recurrence rate and is not recommended as the first technique of choice in patients with constipation.

Transanal approach for the treatment of posterior rectocele is associated with lower resolution of ODS symptoms and a higher recurrence rate with higher infection rates. This approach should be avoided in patients with fecal incontinence or known sphincteric damage, cases in which the association of perineoplasty or levatorplasty may be more indicated.

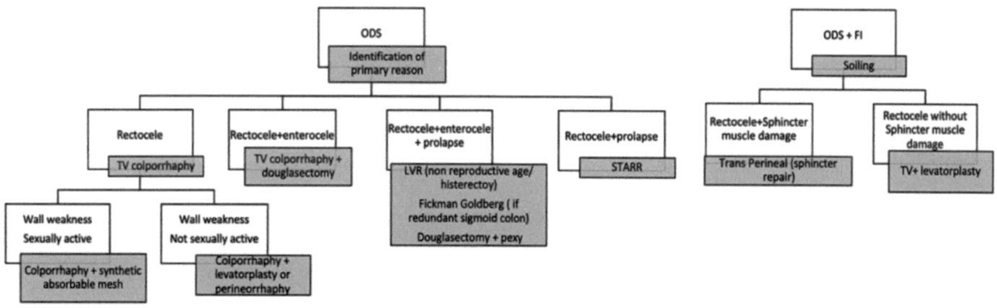

Figure 5.
Option of rectocele treatment algorithm, ODS: Obstructive defecation syndrome, TV: Transvaginal, FI: Fecal incontinence, LVR: Laparoscopic ventral rectopexy, STARR: Stapled transanal rectal resection.

Appendices and nomenclature

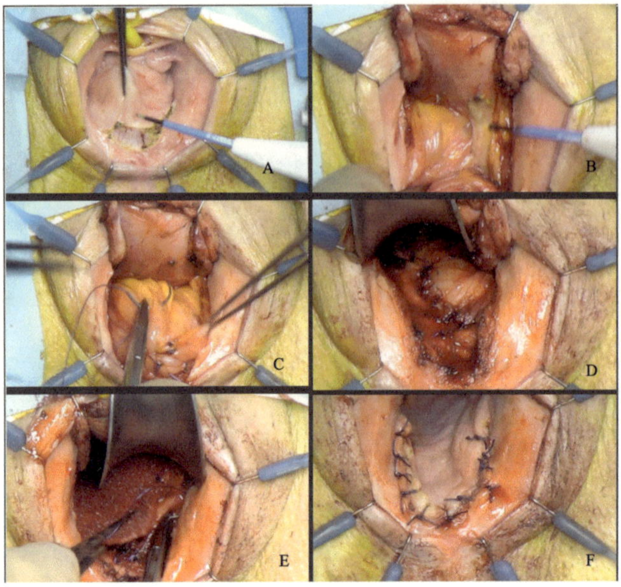

Figure A1.
Transvaginal approach: A. U-shape incision on the vaginal Wall. B. Rectovaginal space dissection. C, D. Plicature (purse string and longitudinal) E. Attachment of the mesh. F Flap closure.

Author details

Esther María Cano Pecharromán*, A. Teresa Calderón Duque, Juan Carlos Santiago Peña and Tomás Balsa Marín
Hospital Nuestra Señora del Prado, Talavera de la Reina, Spain

*Address all correspondence to: esthermcpm@gmail.com

References

[1] Zimmermann EF et al. Transperineal rectocele repair: A systematic review. Royal Australasian College of Surgeons. ANZ Journal of Surgery. 2017;**87**:773-779

[2] Podzemny V, Pescatori LC, Pescatori M. Management of obstructed defecation. World J Gastroenterol. 2015;**21**(4):1053-1060. Available from: http://www.wjgnet.com/1007-9327/full/v21/i4/1053.htm. DOI: 10.3748/wjg.v21.i4.1053

[3] Aubert M, Mege D, Nho R, Meurette G, Sielezneff I. Surgical management of the rectocele- An update. Journal of Visceral Surgery. 2021;**158**(2):145-157

[4] De la Portilla F, García-Armengol J, Espín E, Casal J. AECP (Asociación Española De Coloproctología) Prácticum en Coloproctología de la aecp. Madrid: Ergón; 2022

[5] Brusciano L, Limongelli P, Tolone S, del Genio G, Martellucci J, Docimo G, et al. Technical aspect of stapled transanal rectal resection. From PPH-01 to contour to both. Diseases of the Colon and Rectum. 2015;**58**(8):817-820

[6] García-Mejido JA, Bonomi-Barby MJ, Armijo-Sánchez A, et al. Metodología para el estudio ecográfico transperineal del suelo pélvico. Clínica e Investigación en Ginecología y Obstetricia. 2021;**48**:190-195

[7] Hagen S, Stark D. Conservative prevention and management of pelvic organ prolapse in women. Cochrane Database of Systematic Reviews. 2011;**12**:CD003882

[8] Lacima T, Pera M, Valls-Solé J, González-Argenté X, Puig-Clota M, Espuña M. Electrophysioloigic studies and clinical findings in females with combined fecal and urinary incontinence: A prospective study. Dis Colon Rectum. Mar 2006;**49**(3):353-359. DOI: 10.1007/s10350-005-0277-4. PMID: 16463137

[9] Dietz HP, Wilson PD. Childbirth and pelvic floor trauma. Best Practice & Research Clinical Obstetrics and Gynaecology. 2005;**19**(6):913-924

[10] Tetzschner T et al. Pudendal nerve damage in child birth. Acta Obstetricia et Gynecologica Scandinavica. 2005;**74**:434-440

[11] Chaliha C. Postpartum pelvic floor trauma. Current Opinion in Obstetrics and Gynecology. 2009;**21**:474-479. DOI: 10.1097/GCO.0b013e328332a84e

[12] Manning J et al. The association of obstructive defecation, lower urinary tract dysfunction and the benign joint hypermobility syndrome: A case–control study. International Urogynecological Journal. 2003;**14**:128-132

[13] Balata et al. Transperineal vs. Transanal repair of rectocele. Diseases of the Colon & Rectum. 2020;**63**:4

[14] Grimes CL, Schimpf MO, Wieslander CK, Sleemi A, Doyle P, Wu YM, et al. Surgical interventions for posterior compartment prolapse and obstructed defecation symptoms: A systematic review with clinical practice recommendations. Int Urogynecol J. Sep 2019;**30**(9):1433-1454. DOI: 10.1007/s00192-019-04001-z. Epub 2019 Jun 29. MID: 31256222

[15] Omar W, Elfallal A, Emile S, Elshobaky A, Fouda E, Fathy M, et al.

Horizontal versus vertical plication of the rectovaginal septum in transperineal repair of anterior rectocele: A Pilot Randomized Clinical Trial. Colorectal Disease;**23**(11):3046-3047

[16] Delaini GG, Colucci G. Rectopexy according to Frykman-Goldberg technique. In: Altomare DF, Pucciani F, editors. Rectal Prolapse. Milano: Springer; 2008

[17] Video Correspondence Robotic Frykman–Goldberg procedure for complete rectal prolapse – a video vignette Antonio Sciuto, Raffaele Emmanuele Maria Pirozzi, Alfredo Pede, Gianluca Lanni, Luca Montesarchio, Felice Pirozzi First published: 18 September 2021 https://doi.org/10.1111/codi.15914

[18] Nieminen K, Hiltunen K, Laitinen J, Oksala J, Heinonen P. Transanal or vaginal approach to rectocele repair: A Prospective, Randomized Pilot Study. Diseases of the Colon & Rectum. 2004;**47**(10):1636-1642

[19] Shao Y, Fu Y, Wang Q, Cheng Z, Zhang G, Hu S. Khubchandani's procedure combined with stapled posterior rectal wall resection for rectocele. World Journal of Gastroenterology. 2019;**25**(11):1421-1431

[20] Cruz J, Regadas F, Murad-Regadas S, Rodrigues L, Benicio F, Leal R, et al. TRREMS procedure (transanal repair of rectocele and rectal mucosectomy with one circular stapler): A prospective multicenter trial. Arquivos de Gastroenterologia. 2011;**48**(1):3-7

[21] Gebhart J, Trabuco M. UpToDate. Available from: https://www.uptodate.com/contests/transvaginal-synthetic-mesh-management-of-exposure-and-pain-following-pelvic-sugery?source=related-link. Published 2022

[22] Wein A. Re: FDA Safety Communication: Update on serious complications associated with transvaginal placement of surgical mesh for pelvic organ prolapse. Journal of Urology. 2011;**186**(6):2328-2330

[23] Ribaric G, D'Hoore A, Schiffhorst G, Hempel E. STARR with CONTOUR® TRANSTAR™ device for obstructed defecation syndrome: One-year real-world outcomes of the European TRANSTAR registry. International Journal of Colorectal Disease. 2014;**29**(5):611-622

Chapter 8

Beta-Lactamase-Producing Genes and Integrons in *Escherichia coli* from Diarrheal Children in Ouagadougou, Burkina Faso

René Dembélé, Wendpoulomdé A.D. Kaboré, Issiaka Soulama, Oumar Traoré, Nafissatou Ouédraogo, Ali Konaté, Nathalie K. Guessennd, David Coulibaly N'Golo, Antoine Sanou, Samuel Serme, Soumanaba Zongo, Emmanuel Sampo, Alfred S. Traoré, Amy Gassama-Sow and Nicolas Barro

Abstract

This study aimed to determine the resistance of diarrheagenic *Escherichia coli* (DEC) strains to β-lactams antibiotics and to perform the molecular characterization of extended-spectrum β-lactamases (ESBLs) and integrons genes. It was carried out from August 2013 to October 2015 and involved 31 DEC strains isolated from diarrheal stools samples collected from children less than 5 years. The identification and characterization of DEC strains were done through the standard biochemical tests that were confirmed using API 20E and polymerase chain reaction (PCR). The antibiogram was realized by the disk diffusion method, then an amplification of the β-lactamase resistance genes and integrons by PCR was done. Out of the 419 *E. coli*, 31 isolates (7.4%) harbored the DEC virulence genes. From these DEC, 21 (67.7%) were ESBL-producing *E. coli*. Susceptibility to ESBL-producing *E. coli* showed that the majority of isolates were highly resistant to amoxicillin (77.4%), amoxicillin-clavulanic acid (77.4%), and piperacillin (64.5%). The following antibiotic resistance genes and integron were identified: *bla*TEM (6.5%), *bla*SHV (19.4%), *bla*OXA (38.7%), *bla*CTX-M (9.7%), *Int1* (58.1%), and *Int3* (19.4%). No class 2 integron (*Int2*) was characterized. Because of the high prevalence of multidrug-resistant ESBL organisms found, there is a need of stringent pediatric infection control measures.

Keywords: diarrheagenic, *E. coli*, extended-spectrum β-lactamases, integron, Burkina Faso

1. Introduction

Antimicrobial resistance (AMR) is one of the most serious global public health threats in this century, which is especially urgent regarding antibiotic resistance in bacteria [1], particularly in *Enterobacterales* [2]. This phenomenon has arisen globally in both nosocomial and community settings as a consequence of widespread antibiotics' consumption [3]. *Enterobacterales* are a large order of different types of bacteria including *Escherichia coli* that commonly cause infections both in healthcare settings and in communities [4]. To survive the effects of antibiotics, some *Enterobacterales* can produce enzymes called extended-spectrum β-lactamases (ESBLs) that break down and destroy some commonly used antibiotics, including penicillins and cephalosporins, and make these drugs ineffective for treating infections [4]. Over the last decade, many studies have reported the presence of extended-spectrum β-lactamases (ESBL)-mediated resistance in Gram-negative bacteria causing infections in patients [5–9]. Infections that can be caused by ESBL-producing bacteria include urinary tract infection (UTI), diarrhea, skin infections, and pneumonia [10]. Possible medications used to treat ESBL infection include carbapenems, which are useful against infections caused by *E. coli* or *Klebsiella pneumoniae* bacteria, fosfomycin, β-lactamase inhibitors, non-β-lactam antibiotics, and colistin when other medications have failed to stop the ESBL infection [10]. Unfortunately, the excessive use of antibiotics, in particular β-lactams, leads to the selection of ESBL-producing strains [11]. Because of the emergence and distribution of multidrug-resistant (MDR) *E. coli* is complicating the treatment of various serious infections [12, 13], the World Health Organization (WHO) has long recognized the need for an improved and coordinated global effort to contain AMR [1]. The burden of AMR, including MDR, varies between the regions; however, low- and middle-income countries share a disproportionate burden due to multitude of factors embedded in the characteristics of the health system, policy, and the practice [14].

In Burkina Faso, there is an emergence of β-lactam-resistant enterobacteria, both in rural and urban areas [9, 15–17]. Otherwise, carbapenemase-encoding genes are widespread in many parts of the world [18]. According to a previous study, carbapenemase-producing *Enterobacterales* (CPE) remain one of the most urgent healthcare threats [2]. To this day, the ESBLs and integrons' genes have been poorly characterized in Burkina Faso, particularly in enteric bacteria in children less than 5 years of age. However, it is imperative that bacterial isolates from underdeveloped regions undergo extensive MDR characterization to inform national strategies designed to halt the continuing spread of these dangerous pathogens [19]. Therefore, the aim of this study was to determine the resistance of diarrheagenic *E. coli* strains to β-lactams antibiotics and perform the molecular characterization of extended-spectrum β-lactamases (ESBL) and integrons genes among clinical DEC isolated from stools collected in children less than 5 years of age.

2. Methodology

2.1 Study design, area, and sample population

It is a cross-sectional study conducted in two hospitals of Ouagadougou, Burkina Faso (Paul VI and Schiphra), during August 2013 to October 2015 (**Figure 1**). The Paul VI hospital is located in peripheral area and the Schiphra's hospital in the city

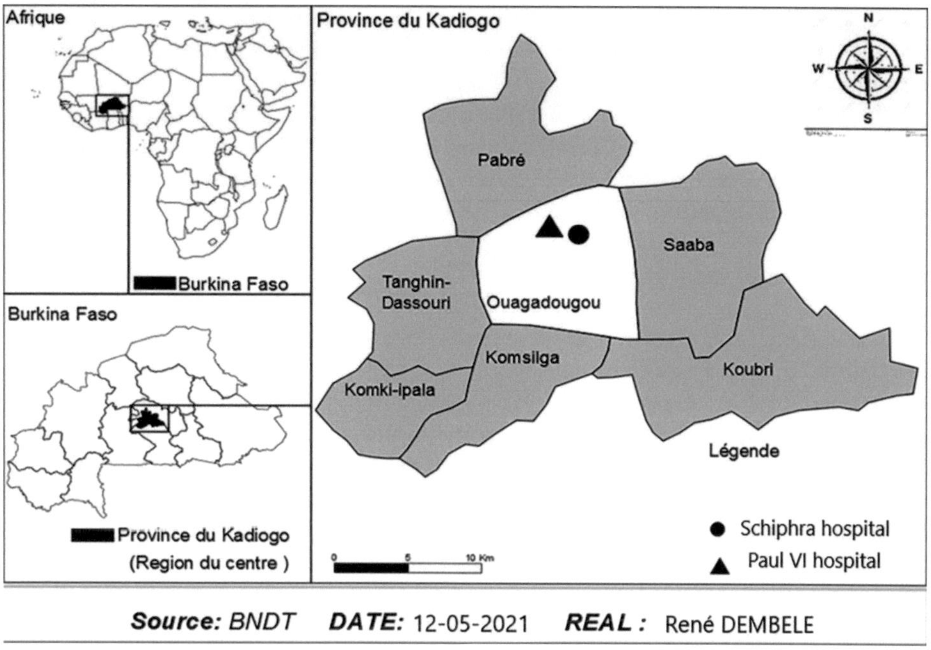

Figure 1.
Sampling sites in Ouagadougou.

center at the dam edge of Ouagadougou. Many patients from Ouagadougou and its surroundings attend these two healthcare centers because of the good level of healthcare. The study population comprised children below 5 years attending the hospital for treatment.

The specimens were collected adhering to a standard protocol from pediatric patients below 5 years of age with acute diarrhea and who were hospitalized or visited the health centers as outpatient. Thus, children who attended the hospitals for treatment and provided assent (from parents) or consent for the study were included in the study. Any child over the age of 5 years was excluded from the study.

2.2 Sample collection and transport

Three hundred and fifteen stool samples were collected in sterile containers and transported to the laboratory of molecular biology, epidemiology, and surveillance of bacteria and viruses transmitted by food, center for research in biological, food, and nutritional sciences at the Joseph KI-ZERBO University of Ouagadougou within 24 h in a cool box at +4°C for immediate analysis.

2.3 Bacterial isolates

Isolation of *E. coli* was carried out onto eosin methylene blue agar (Liofilchem, Italy), and the plates were incubated at +37°C for 18–24 h. After this stage, the suspected *E. coli* colonies were selected and streaked onto Mueller-Hinton agar plate (Liofilchem, Italy). Confirmation was carried out by a biochemical microbiology method based on negative urease (Bio-Rad, France), negative citrate (Liofilchem, Italy), positive indole (Bio-Rad, France), positive lactose (Liofilchem, Italy), and positive orthonitrophenyl-β-D-galactopyranoside (ONPG) (bioMerieux, France). *E. coli* strains isolated were confirmed by API 20E (bioMérieux, France).

The five main pathogroups of *E. coli* (Enteroaggregative *E. coli:* EAEC, Enteropathogenic *E. coli*: EPEC, Enteroinvasive *E. coli*: EIEC, Enterohemorrhagic *E. coli*: EHEC, and Enterotoxigenic *E. coli*: ETEC) were characterized by the 16-plex polymerase chain reaction (PCR) as described by Antikainen et al. [20].

2.4 Antimicrobial susceptibility testing

All identified isolates of *E. coli* were treated for susceptibility testing against amoxicillin (25 µg), amoxicillin-clavulanic acid (20/10 µg), ceftriaxone (30 µg), cefotaxime (30 µg), cefepime (30 µg), cefixime (10 µg), piperacillin (75 µg), piperacillin-tazobactam (100 + 10 µg), imipenem (10 µg), and aztreonam (30 µg) (Bio-Rad, France) following disk diffusion method on Mueller-Hinton Agar (Liofilchem, Italy). Results were interpreted based on the European Committee of Antimicrobial Susceptibility Testing (EUCAST) guidelines [21]. These isolates, which were not susceptible (either resistant or intermediate) to three or more antibiotics classes, were considered as MDR [22].

2.5 Screening and confirmation of ESBL and integrons producers

A double synergy test was used for ESBL-producing strains testing. This consisted of placing disks (2–3 cm diameter) of ceftriaxone and cefotaxime around an amoxicillin-clavulanic acid disk on the bacterial plate.

For molecular characterization, DNA extraction was performed using heating method [23]. A loopful of bacterial growth from Mueller-Hinton agar (Liofilchem, Italy) plate was suspended in 1 ml of sterilized water. The mixture was boiled for 10 min at +100°C and centrifuged for 10 min at 12000 rpm at +4°C. Supernatant was then collected and used for the PCR reactions as DNA matrices. Multiplex PCR assays were performed for detecting EBLS-encoding genes (bla_{TEM}, bla_{SHV}, bla_{OXA}, and $bla_{\text{CTX-M}}$) and the presence of the class 1, class 2, and class 3 integrons from the β-lactams-resistant DEC strains. Primers (GeneCust, France) used for these amplifications are described in **Table 1**.

Thermocycling conditions were as follows: 5 min at +94°C, followed by 35 amplification cycles of +94°C for 30 s, 59 ± 4°C for 60 s, and +72°C for 60 s with a final extension of +72°C for 10 min on a thermal cycler (Gene Amp 9700, Applied Biosystems). PCR products were revealed on 1.5% stained Redsaf agarose gel (Prolabo, France), after electrophoresis under UV light (Gel Logic 200).

The PCR assays were carried out in a 25-ml reaction mixture, which consisted of 2.5 µl of the supernatant added to 22.5 µl of reaction mixture. This mixture contained 5 U of Taq DNA polymerase (Accu Power, South Korea), deoxyribonucleic triphosphate (10 mM), buffer GC (10X), $MgCl_2$ (25 mM), and PCR primers (10 µM). Thermocycling conditions were as follows: 5 min at +94°C, followed by 35 amplification cycles at +94°C for 30 s, + 59 ± 4°C for 60 s, and +72°C for 60 s with a final extension of +72°C for 10 min on a thermal cycler (AB Applied Biosystems). Following PCR, the reaction products were separated using electrophoresis in 1.5% agarose gel (weight/volume), stained with Redsaf solution (Prolabo, France), and visualized under UV light (Gel Logic 200) [23].

Genetic resistance supports	Genes	Primers sequence (5′ to 3′)	Product size (bp)
β-Lactams resistance gene	*bla*$_{TEM}$	F: ATG AGT ATT CAA CAT TTC CG	1080
		R: CCA ATG CTT ATT CAG TGA GG	
	bla$_{SHV}$	F: TTA TCT CCC TGT TAG CCA CC	768
		R: GAT TTG CTG ATT TCG CTC GG	
	bla$_{OXA}$	F: ATG AAA AAC ACA ATA CAT ATC	813
		R: AAT TTA GTG TGT TTA GAA TGG	
	bla$_{CTX-M}$	F: -ATG TGC AGY ACC AGT AAR GT	544
		R: -TGG GTR AAR TAR GTS ACC AGA	
Integrons	*Int1*	F: ATT TCT GTC CTG GCT GGC GA	600
		R: ACA TGT GAT GGC GAC GCA CGA	
	Int2	F: CAC GGA TAT GCG ACA AAA AGG T	806
		R: GTA GCA AAC GAC TGA CGA AAT G	
	Int3	F: GCC CCG GCA GCG ACT TTC AG	600
		R: ACG GCT CTG CCA AAC CTG ACT	

Table 1.
List of all primers used for antibiotic ESBL genes and integrons detection.

2.6 Statistical analysis

The Fisher's exact test with two-tailed p of Open Epi version 7.1.2.0 was used to determine the statistical significance of the results. A p value of <0.05 was considered statistically significant.

3. Results

3.1 Prevalence of bacterial isolates

From 315 children with diarrhea, 192 stool samples were positive to one suspected *E. coli* detection (60.9%). Four hundred and nineteen (419) strains of *E. coli* were isolated, from which 31 DEC (7.4%) were characterized. From these DEC, 21 DEC were ESBL-producing *E. coli* (67.7%).

3.2 Antimicrobial susceptibility

All the DEC strains tested for the 10 β-lactams antibiotics showed important resistances to the aminopenicillins. However, few cephalosporins and carbapenems were yet active on some pathotypes (**Table 2**).

3.3 Correlation between resistance phenotype and resistance genetic supports

Nineteen (19) out of the 21 ESBLs-producing *E. coli* (90.5%) had ESBLs genes. The following resistance genes were characterized: 12 *bla*$_{OXA}$ (38.7%), 6 *bla*$_{SHV}$ (19.4%),

β-Lactams subfamilies	Antibiotics	Prevalence of antibiotic susceptibility N (%)		DEC resistance prevalence N (%)				
		Resistant	Sensitive	EPEC ($n = 8$)	EHEC ($n = 3$)	EIEC ($n = 4$)	EAEC ($n = 15$)	ETEC ($n = 1$)
Penicillins	Amoxicillin	24 (77.4)	7 (22.6)	6 (76)	2 (66.6)	4 (100)	11 (73.3)	1 (100)
	Amoxicillin-clavulanic acid	24 (77.4)	7 (22.6)	6 (76)	2 (66.6)	4 (100)	11 (73.3)	1 (100)
	Piperacillin	20 (64.5)	11 (35.5)	5 (62.5)	2 (66.6)	3 (75)	9 (60)	1 (100)
	Piperacillin-tazobactam	12 (38.7)	19 (61.3)	3 (37.5)	2 (66.6)	1 (25)	5 (33.3)	1 (100)
Cephalosporins	Ceftriaxone	13 (41.9)	18 (58.1)	2 (25)	1 (33.3)	2 (50)	7 (46.6)	1 (100)
	Cefixime	13 (41.9)	18 (58.1)	2 (25)	1 (33.3)	2 (50)	7 (46.6)	1 (100)
	Cefotaxim	14 (45.2)	17 (54.8)	2 (25)	2 (66.6)	2 (50)	7 (46.6)	1 (100)
	Cefepim	14 (45.2)	17 (54.8)	2 (25)	2 (66.6)	2 (50)	7 (46.6)	1 (100)
Monobactam	Aztreonam	14 (45.2)	17 (54.8)	2 (25)	2 (66.6)	2 (50)	7 (46.6)	1 (100)
Carbapenems	Imipenem	5 (16.1)	26 (83.9)	1 (12.5)	1 (33.3)	0 (0)	3 (20)	0 (0)

Table 2.
Antimicrobials susceptibility of the studied isolates to β-lactams.

DEC strains	Resistance phenotypes	Antibiotics										Genetic resistance supports						
												Resistance genes				Integrons		
		AMC	AMX	CTX	ATM	IPM	CRO	FEP	CFM	TZP	PIP	bla_{TEM}	bla_{SHV}	bla_{OXA}	bla_{CTX-M}	*IntI1*	*IntI2*	*IntI3*
Schiphra's hospital (*n* = 9/18; 50%)																		
EHEC	ESBL, Carbapenemase	R	R	R	R	R	-	R	-	R	R	-	+	+	+	+	-	-
aEPEC	ESBL	R	R	-	-	-	-	-	-	-	-	+	-	-	-	+	-	-
tEPEC	ESBL	R	R	R	R	-	R	R	R	R	R	-	-	+	-	+	-	-
tEPEC	ESBL	R	R	-	-	-	-	-	-	R	R	-	+	-	-	+	-	-
EIEC	ESBL	R	R	-	-	-	-	-	-	-	R	-	+	-	-	+	-	+
EAEC	ESBL	R	R	-	-	-	-	-	-	-	R	-	+	-	-	+	-	-
EAEC	ESBL	R	R	-	-	-	-	-	-	-	-	-	+	-	-	+	-	-
EAEC	ESBL, Carbapenemase	R	R	R	R	R	R	R	R	R	R	-	-	-	+	+	-	-
EAEC	ESBL	R	R	R	R	-	R	R	R	R	R	-	-	+	-	+	-	-
Paul VI hospital (n = 10/13; 76.9%)																		
aEPEC	ESBL, PHN	R	R	-	-	-	-	-	-	-	R	-	-	+	-	+	-	-
aEPEC	ESBL, Carbapenemase	R	R	R	R	R	R	R	R	R	R	-	-	+	-	+	-	-
aEPEC	ESBL, PHN	R	R	-	-	-	-	-	-	-	R	-	-	+	-	+	-	-
EIEC	ESBL, PHN	R	R	R	R	-	R	R	R	R	R	-	+	+	-	-	-	+
EAEC	ESBL, PHN	R	R	-	-	-	-	-	-	-	R	-	-	+	-	+	-	-
ETEC	CASE, PHN	R	R	R	R	-	R	R	R	R	R	-	-	+	-	+	-	-
EAEC	ESBL, PHN	R	R	-	-	-	-	-	-	-	R	-	-	+	-	+	-	-

DEC strains	Resistance phenotypes	Antibiotics										Genetic resistance supports						
												Resistance genes				Integrons		
		AMC	AMX	CTX	ATM	IPM	CRO	FEP	CFM	TZP	PIP	*bla*$_{TEM}$	*bla*$_{SHV}$	*bla*$_{OXA}$	*bla*$_{CTX-M}$	*IntI1*	*IntI2*	*IntI3*
EAEC	ESBL, PBN	R	R	R	R	-	R	R	R	-	S	+	-	-	-	+	-	-
EAEC	ESBL, Carbapenemase	R	R	R	R	R	R	R	R	R	R	-	-	+	+	+	-	-
EAEC	ESBL	R	R	R	R	-	R	R	R	-	-	-	-	+	-	+	-	-

EAEC = Enteroaggregative E. coli, aEPEC = Atypical Enteropathogenic E. coli, tEPEC = Typical Enteropathogenic E. coli, EIEC = Enteroinvasive E. coli, EHEC = Enterohemorrhagic E. coli, ETEC = Enterotoxigenic E. coli, PHN = High-level penicillinases, CASE = Cephalosporinases, ESBL = Extended-spectrum β-lactamases, AMC = Amoxicillin-Clavulanic Acid, AMX = Amoxicillin, CTX = Cefotaxime, ATM = Aztreonam, IPM = Imipenem, CRO = Ceftriaxone, FEP = Cefepime, CFM = Cefixime, TZP = Piperacillin-tazobactam, PIP = Piperacillin, R = Resistant, − = Absence, + = Presence.

Table 3.
Correlation between E. coli pathotypes, antibiotics resistance, and genetic resistance supports.

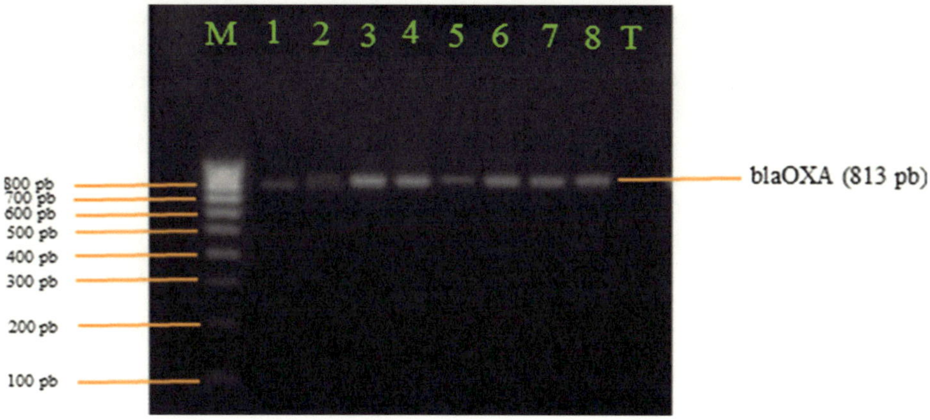

Figure 2.
bla_{OXA} gene on agarose gel electrophoresis (1.5%). Lane M: molecular size marker (100 bp), 1: bla_{OXA1}: positive control (813 pb), lanes: 2–8 are positive for bla_{OXA} gene, lane T: negative control.

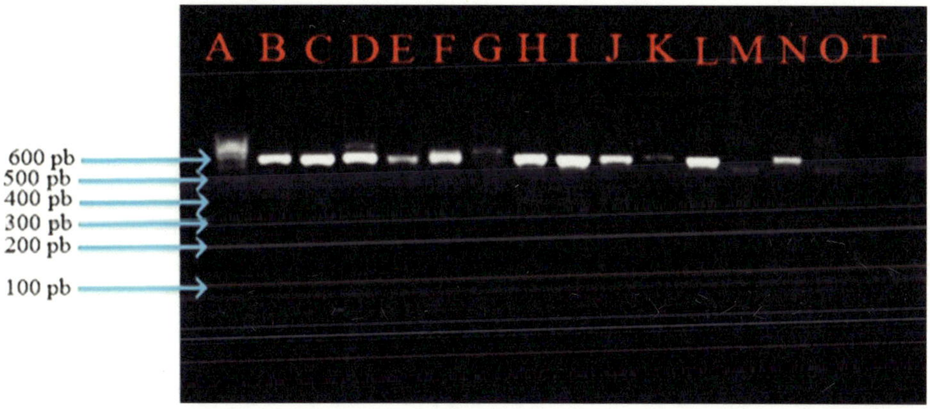

Figure 3.
Int1 gene on agarose gel electrophoresis (1.5%). Lane A: molecular size marker (100 bp), B: Int1: positive control (600 pb), lanes: C-O are positive for Int1 gene, lane T: negative control.

3 $bla_{CTX\text{-}M}$ (9.7%), and 2 bla_{TEM} (6.5%). Our results showed that the genes responsible for the production of bla_{OXA} β-lactamases 12/31 (38.7%) were more prevalent in comparison to the genes encoding bla_{TEM}, bla_{SHV}, and $bla_{CTX\text{-}M}$ β-lactamases (**Table 3**). From the three classes of integrons (*Int1, Int2*, and *Int3*) assessed among the resistant strains carrying ESBL genes, only 18 *Int1* (58.1%) and 2 *Int3* (19.4%) were detected. The class 3 integron was detected in only EIEC. No class 2 integrons (*Int2*) were characterized from the resistant strains. The coexistence of the three resistance genes (bla_{SHV}, bla_{OXA}, and $bla_{CTX\text{-}M}$) and *Int1* was found in one EHEC (**Table 3**). The bla_{OXA} gene (**Figure 2**) was associated with *Int1* (**Figure 3**) in 11 cases (p = 0.001), while the bla_{SHV} gene was associated with *Int1* in 5 cases (p = 0.100).

4. Discussion

The emergence and spread of multidrug-resistant (MDR) bacteria are major public health threats worldwide. Particularly, DEC that produce ESBL are of great concern, because their resistance to penicillins and narrow extended-spectrum cephalosporins reduces considerably the treatment options. The prevalence of ESBL in *Enterobacteriaceae* has been detected at local levels in various African countries; moreover, a study was conducted in 2014 on the prevalence of ESBL and what type of genes are involved in its occurrence [24]. The frequency of ESBL-producing *E. coli* was 67.7% in our study. Similar prevalence was reported in Egypt (69.6%) [25] and Palestine (66.7%) [26]. Nevertheless, our prevalence was higher than those in Burkina Faso (58%) [6], Iran (40.8%) [27], Saudi Arabia (30.6%) [28], Japan (20.4%) [29], Colombia (11.7%) [30], and Nepal (22.7%) [31]. Otherwise, our result is lower than the ESBL production in clinical isolates of *E. coli* reported somewhere else in Iran [32]. The prevalence of ESBL resistance in *E. coli* isolates in European countries is reported to be around 3.9% with variations between countries [33]. Overall, these percentages are lower than those found in middle-income countries like Thailand (71.25%) [34] and China (50.5%) [35]. This difference between ESBLs' prevalence might be due to patient's age, the type of samples, and the country health facilities in the management of diarrheal infections regarding antibiotics use. Indeed, in developing countries, most patients received antibiotics treatment without prescription [36, 37]; such common practices in nearly all developing countries cause a selective pressure on *E. coli*, whereas in more developed countries effective strategies for the control of antimicrobial are present, which effectively prevents the emergence of ESBLs [36].

It has been reported that bacteria such as *E. coli* and *K. pneumoniae* are major ESBL producers resulting in serious threat to the treatment regimen [38]. Indeed, ESBL enzymes are becoming increasingly expressed by many strains of pathogenic bacteria presenting diagnostic challenges to the clinical microbiology laboratories [39, 40]. Until recently, antimicrobial therapy has played an important role in the treatment of human bacterial infections. However, the drug resistance has emerged in the treatment of bacterial infections due to ESBL enzymes [39]. Indeed, these enzymes can degrade all β-lactam antibiotics leading to multidrug-resistant bacteria. Therefore, reporting of ESBL-producing isolates from clinical samples is critical for the clinicians. It constitutes the guidelines to select appropriate antibiotics for the treatment, including to take proper precaution to prevent the spread of these resistant organisms to other patients [31].

The present study shows 19 ESBLs genes (90.5%) out of the 21 ESBLs-producing *E. coli*. Analysis of the ESBL-encoding genes indicated that the majority of the ESBL-positive isolates harbored bla_{OXA} (38.7%), followed by bla_{SHV} (19.4%), $bla_{\mathrm{CTX\text{-}M}}$ (9.7%), and bla_{TEM} (6.5%). The emergence of β-lactam resistance in *Enterobacteriaceae* is related primarily to the production of enzymes such as TEM and SHV variant, which were the most common ESBLs during the past decade. However, OXA and CTX-M β-lactamases have emerged as prevalent ESBL worldwide type compared with the TEM and SHV genotypes [41].

In the present study, OXA-type ESBL-producing DEC strains (38.7%) were the most frequently detected ESBL gene. This prevalence is lower than that reported in our previous study in rural area of Burkina Faso: 100% [9], also lower comparatively to 52% reported in Pakistan [42]. However, a recent study in young children reported 3% of commensal *E. coli* bearing the bla_{OXA} gene in Bangladesh [41]. Thus, it appears that the emergence of ESBLs-producing bacteria among gut bacteria of young children can transfer resistance and related genes horizontally across pathogenic *E. coli*, and commensal *E. coli* leading to a public health concern. Most of the OXA-type ESBL-producing *E. coli* isolates (29%) in our study were detected from the Paul VI hospital (p = 0.002). This hospital is located in peripheral area of Ouagadougou, and most of the people living in the slums with poor sanitation conditions attend it for healthcare sought. Moreover, the provision of confessional care has less difficult accessibility for the peripheral neighborhoods and the population with low socioeconomic level. Otherwise, people in Burkina Faso do not consult a healthcare agent in the case of diseases such as gastrointestinal infections and use self-medication instead [37]. Our results showed 19.4% of SHV-type ESBL-producing *E. coli* which is a little similar to 21% detected in Pakistan [42]. By cons, this prevalence is higher than 0% [9] and 5.9% [17], previously reported in Burkina Faso but lower than 45% reported in Iran [27]. The $bla_{\text{CTX-M}}$ gene (**Figure 4**) has been detected in three *E. coli* isolates, while its prevalence was 25% in our earlier report [9] and 40.1% by a study conducted in *Enterobacteriaceae* from Burkinabe patients [17]. Moreover, few studies from other parts of world have shown different prevalence of $bla_{\text{CTX-M}}$ gene among isolates, including 98.8% (China), 84.7% (Chile), 13.6% (Tanzania), 76% (Pakistan), 97.8% (Chad), and 81.6% (Egypt) [25, 42–46]. Indeed, CTX-M β-lactamases are recognized as the most widespread extended-spectrum β-lactamases (ESBLs) among clinical isolates of *Enterobacteriaceae* [47]. Besides, an earlier report from Nigeria has shown the predominance of CTX-M15 in wild birds and cattle in Nigeria [48] suggesting that this gene could be transferred to humans by animals. Finally, our study revealed 6.5% of TEM-type ESBL-producing *E. coli*, while no bla_{TEM} gene has been detected in our previous study [9]. However, this value is lower than 26.2 and 28% reported in Burkina Faso and Pakistan, respectively [17, 42]. The resistance to amoxicillin/amoxicillin-clavulanic acid observed in the two *E. coli* strains (6.5%) may be mainly mediated by the production of these plasmid-encoded TEM enzymes.

Among the three class of integron, class 1 integron (58.1%) was majority characterized from the resistant strains in accordance with 56% reported in Bangladesh [41]. This result confirms those of previous studies showing that class 1 integron was predominantly represented in *Enterobacteriaceae* [49, 50]. However, a previous report in Burkina Faso has shown a lower prevalence (44.4%) of *Int1* [51]. On the other hand, studies reported a high prevalence of *Int1* (80%) in *E. coli* isolated from dairy products consumed in Burkina Faso [52] and in human, animal, and food in Spain [53]. This could increase the risk of emergence and spread of MDR *E. coli*, since humans are always in contact with these

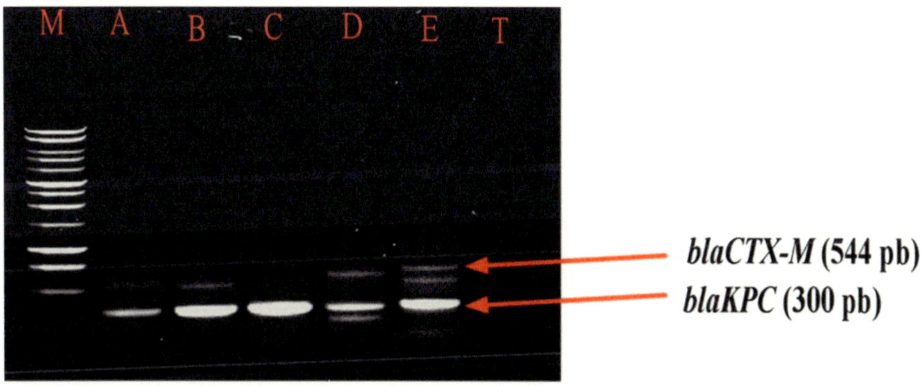

Figure 4.
$bla_{\text{CTX-M}}$ gene on agarose gel electrophoresis (1.5%). Lane M: molecular size marker (100 bp), A: $bla_{\text{CTX-M}}$ positive control (544 pb), lanes: B, D, and E are positive for $bla_{\text{CTX-M}}$ gene (544 pb), lane T: negative control.

different ecosystems, especially when there is a lack of food hygiene and sanitation. Moreover, class 1 integrons can facilitate the spread of antibiotic-resistant genes meaning that it could have public health consequences [54].

The class 3 integron was detected in only EIEC. No class 2 integron (*Int2*) was characterized from the resistant strains. By cons, 22.2% of *Int2* was detected in our previous study [51]. Moreover, a study also found the presence of *Int2* gene in Senegalese *Shigella* spp. isolates [49].

Two strains of EIEC harbored both class 1 and 3 integrons. However, a previous study showed that *E. coli* harbored class 1 and 2 integrons simultaneously [50]. Otherwise, in the present study, one EIEC strain was resistant to aztreonam and imipenem and possesses ESBL-carbapenemase phenotype. This strain was resistant to all subfamilies (penicillins, cephalosporins, monobactam, and carbapenems) of β-lactams antibiotic tested and also showed simultaneous presence of bla_{SHV}, bla_{OXA}, $bla_{CTX\text{-}M}$, and *Int1*. Indeed, strains that had this aztreonam-resistant phenotype possessed both the resistance gene [27]. Resistance to this antibiotic could be explained by genetic mutations [43]. It has been described that the coexistence of these two classes of integrons [42] and/or several genes suggests that they have integrated the same gene and give these strains a high level of resistance. However, bla_{TEM}, bla_{SHV}, bla_{OXA}, $bla_{CTX\text{-}M}$ as well as integrons (*Int1, Int2, and Int3*) are involved in the antibiotic resistance of DEC, but the presence of resistant strains producing ESBL and lacking ESBL gene (bla_{TEM}, bla_{SHV}, bla_{OXA}, and $bla_{CTX\text{-}M}$) and integron suggests that there are other mechanisms for the dissemination of antibiotic resistance in DEC strains.

5. Conclusion

This study highlights the important involvement of genes and integrons into multidrug resistance strains of *E. coli* in two main hospitals of Ouagadougou. The most important finding was the detection of four *E. coli* multiresistant strains producing ESBL that were resistant to imipenem, aztreonam, and harbored class 1 integrons. Another important observation was the detection of two *E. coli* multiresistant strains producing ESBL but lacking a resistance gene and/or integrons. Our results have demonstrated the emergence and dissemination of multidrug-resistant *E. coli* strains hosting several genes responsible for the production of ESBL in clinical isolates. Ultimately, to fight effectively against the emergence of antimicrobial resistance, an integrated surveillance network should be set up, which would be of great benefit to national antimicrobial resistance control programs.

Acknowledgements

The authors gratefully thank "Réseau de Recherche sur les Maladies Entériques à potentiel épidémique en Afrique de l'Ouest (REMENTA)/Programme d'Appui à la Recherche en Réseau en Afrique (PARRAF)" for technical support. The authors also thank the parents and guardians of children as well as the authorities of the Paul VI and Schiphra's hospitals for their honest cooperation.

Author details

René Dembélé[1,2]*, Wendpoulomdé A.D. Kaboré[1], Issiaka Soulama[3], Oumar Traoré[1,2], Nafissatou Ouédraogo[1,2], Ali Konaté[1,†], Nathalie K. Gucssennd[4,5], David Coulibaly N'Golo[5], Antoine Sanou[3], Samuel Serme[3], Soumanaba Zongo[3], Emmanuel Sampo[6], Alfred S. Traoré[1], Amy Gassama-Sow[7,†] and Nicolas Barro[1]

1 Laboratory of Molecular Biology, Epidemiology and Surveillance of Bacteria and Viruses Transmitted by Food, Centre for Research in Biological, Food and Nutritional Sciences, Graduate School of Sciences and Technologies, Joseph KI-ZERBO University, Ouagadougou, Burkina Faso

2 Training and Research Unit in Applied Sciences and Technologies, University of Dedougou, Dedougou, Burkina Faso

3 National Centre for Research and Training on Malaria, Ouagadougou, Burkina Faso

4 Laboratory of Bacteriology-Virology, Unit of Antibiotics, Natural Substances and Surveillance of Resistance of Microorganisms to Antimicrobials, Pasteur Institute of Abidjan, Abidjan, Ivory Coast

5 Laboratory of Bacteriology-Virology, Unit of Training and Research of Medical Sciences, University Felix Houphouet BOIGNY, Abidjan, Ivory Coast

6 Schiphra's Hospital, Ouagadougou, Burkina Faso

7 Unit of Experimental Bacteriology, Pasteur Institute of Dakar, Dakar, Senegal

*Address all correspondence to: simavedemb@gmail.com

† Ali Konaté and Amy Gassama-Sow are deceased.

References

[1] Prestinaci F, Pezzotti P, Pantosti A. Antimicrobial resistance: A global multifaceted phenomenon. Pathogens and Global Health. 2015;**109**(7):309-318

[2] Dembélé R, Soulama I, Kaboré WAD, Konaté A, Kagambèga A, Coulibaly DN, et al. Molecular characterization of carbapenemase-producing *Enterobacterales* in children with diarrhea in rural Burkina Faso. Journal of Drug Delivery and Therapeutics. 2021;**11**(1):84-92

[3] Ashley EA, Lubell Y, White NJ, Turner P. Antimicrobial susceptibility of bacterial isolates from community acquired infections in Sub-Saharan Africa and Asian low and middle income countries. Tropical Medicine & International Health. 2011;**16**:1167-1169

[4] Centers for Disease Control and Prevention, National Center for Emerging and Zoonotic Infectious Diseases (NCEZID), Division of Healthcare Quality Promotion (DHQP). Healthcare-Associated Infections (HAI), Diseases and Organisms. 2019

[5] Raut S, Gokhale S, Adhikari B. Prevalence of extended spectrum beta-lactamases among *E. coli* and *Klebsiella* spp isolates in Manipal, Teaching Hospital, Pokhara, Nepal. Journal of Microbiology and Infectious Diseases. 2015;5:69-75

[6] Ouédraogo AS, Sanou M, Kissou A, Sanou S, Solaré H, Kaboré F, et al. High prevalence of extended-spectrum β-lactamase producing *Enterobacteriaceae* among clinical isolates in Burkina Faso. BMC Infectious Diseases. 2016;**16**:326

[7] Nepal K, Pant ND, Neupane B, Belbase A, Baidhya R, Shrestha RK, et al. Extended spectrum beta-lactamase and metallo beta-lactamase production among *Escherichia coli* and *Klebsiella pneumoniae* isolated from different clinical samples in a tertiary care hospital in Kathmandu, Nepal. Annals of Clinical Microbiology and Antimicrobials. 2017;**16**:62

[8] Rai S, Pant ND, Bhandari R, Giri A, Parajuli R, Aryal M, et al. AmpC and extended spectrum beta-lactamases production among urinary isolates from a tertiary care hospital in Lalitpur, Nepal. BMC Research Notes. 2017;**10**:467

[9] Dembélé R, Konaté A, Traoré O, Kaboré WAD, Soulama I, Kagambèga A, et al. Extended spectrum beta-lactamase and fluoroquinolone resistance genes among *Escherichia coli* and *Salmonella* isolates from children with diarrhea, Burkina Faso. BMC Pediatrics. 2020a;**20**:459

[10] Jewell T, Biggers A. ESBLs (Extended Spectrum Beta-Lactamases). 2017. Available from: https://www.healthline.com/health/esbl [Updated: 14 April]

[11] Chang YT, Coombs G, Ling T, Balaji V, Rodrigues C, Mikamo H, et al. Epidemiology and trends in the antibiotic susceptibilities of Gram negative bacilli isolated from patients with intra-abdominal infections in the Asia-Pacific region, 2010-2013. International Journal of Antimicrobial Agents. 2017;**49**:734-739

[12] Allocati N, Masulli M, Alexeyev MF, Ilio CD. *Escherichia coli* in Europe: An overview. International Journal of Environmental Research and Public Health. 2013;**10**:6235-6254

[13] Mariappan S, Sekar U, Kamalanathan A. Carbapenemase-producing *Enterobacteriaceae*: Risk factors for infection and impact of resistance on outcomes. International Journal of Applied & Basic Medical Research. 2018;7:32-39

[14] Pokharel S, Raut S, Adhikari B. Tackling antimicrobial resistance in low- and middle-income countries. BMJ Global Health. 2019;**4**:e002104

[15] Dembélé R, Bonkoungou IJO, Konaté A, Bsadjo-Tchamba G, Bawa HI, Bako E, et al. Serotyping and antibiotic resistance of enteropathogenic *Escherichia coli* and *E. coli* O157 isolated from diarrheal children in rural area of Burkina Faso. African Journal of Microbiology Research. 2015;**9**:1053-1059

[16] Ouédraogo A-S, Sanou S, Kissou A, Poda A, Aberkane S, Bouzinbi N, et al. Fecal carriage of *Enterobacteriaceae* producing extended-spectrum beta-lactamases in hospitalized patients and healthy community volunteers in Burkina Faso. Microbial Drug Resistance. 2017;**23**:1

[17] Kpoda DS, Ajayi A, Somda M, Traore O, Guessennd N, Ouattara AS, et al. Distribution of resistance genes encoding ESBLs in *Enterobacteriaceae* isolated from biological samples in health centers in Ouagadougou, Burkina Faso. BMC Research Notes. 2018;**11**:471

[18] Halat DH, Moubareck CA. The current burden of carbapenemases: Review of significant properties and dissemination among gram-negative bacteria. Antibiotica. 2020;**9**:186

[19] Margulieux KR, Srijan A, Ruekit S, Nobthai P, Poramathikul K, Pandey P, et al. Extended-spectrum β-lactamase prevalence and virulence factor characterization of enterotoxigenic *Escherichia coli* responsible for acute diarrhea in Nepal from 2001 to 2016. Antimicrobial Resistance and Infection Control. 2018;7:87

[20] Antikainen J, Tarkka E, Haukka K, Siitonen A, Vaara M, Kirveskari J. New 16 plex PCR method for rapid detection of diarrheagenic *Escherichia coli* directly from stool samples. European Journal of Clinical Microbiology & Infectious Diseases. 2009;**28**:899-908

[21] European Committee on Antimicrobial Susceptibility Testing (EUCAST). Recommandation 2017. Éd. V.1.0 Mars. 2017. pp. 1-127. Available from: https://www.eucast.org/

[22] Magiorakos AP, Srinivasan A, Carey RB, Carmeli Y, Falagas ME, Giske CG, et al. Multidrug-resistant, extensively drug-resistant and pandrug-resistant bacteria: An international expert proposal for interim standard definitions for acquired resistance. Clinical Microbiology and Infection. 2012;**18**:268-281

[23] Moyo SJ, Maselle SY, Matee MI, Langeland N, Mylvaganam H. Identification of diarrheagenic *Escherichia coli* isolated from infants and children in Dar es Salaam, Tanzania. BMC Infectious Diseases. 2007;7(92):1-7

[24] Storberg V. ESBL-producing *Enterobacteriaceae* in Africa—A non-systematic literature review of research published 2008-2012. Infection Ecology & Epidemiology. 2014;**4**(1):20342

[25] Mohamed ES, Khairy RMM, Abdelrahim SS. Prevalence and molecular characteristics of ESBL and AmpC β-lactamase producing *Enterobacteriaceae* strains isolated from UTIs in Egypt. Antimicrobial Resistance and Infection Control. 2020;**9**:198

[26] Tayh G, Laham NA, Yahia HB, Sallem RB, Elottol AE, Slama KB. Extended-spectrum β-lactamases among enterobacteriaceae isolated from urinary tract infections in Gaza Strip, Palestine. BioMed Research International. 2019. Article ID: 4041801,11

[27] Seyedjavadi SS, Goudarzi M, Sabzehali F. Relation between bla_{TEM}, bla_{SHV} and bla_{CTX-M} genes and acute urinary tract infections. Journal of Acute Diseases. 2016;**5**:71-76

[28] Hassan H, Abdalhamid B. Molecular characterization of extended spectrum beta-lactamase producing *Enterobacteriaceae* in a Saudi Arabian tertiary hospital. Journal of Infection in Developing Countries. 2014;**8**:282-288

[29] Harada Y, Morinaga Y, Yamada K, Migiyama Y, Nagaoka K, Uno N, et al. Clinical and molecular epidemiology of extended spectrum β-lactamase-producing *Klebsiella pneumoniae* and *Escherichia coli* in a Japanese tertiary hospital. Journal of Medical Microbiology and Diagnosis. 2013;**2**:127

[30] Martinez P, Garzôn D, Mattar S. CTX-M-producing *Escherichia coli* and *Klebsiella pneumoniae* isolated from community-acquired urinary tract infections in Valledupar, Colombia. Brazilian Journal of Infectious Diseases. 2012;**16**:420-425

[31] Kayastha K, Dhungel B, Karki S, Adhikari B, Banjara MR, Rijal KR, et al. Extended-spectrum β-lactamase-producing *Escherichia coli* and *Klebsiella* species in pediatric patients visiting International Friendship Children's Hospital, Kathmandu, Nepal. Infectious Diseases: Research and Treatment. 2020;**13**:1-7

[32] Najar PS, Eslami M, Memariani M, Siadat SD. High prevalence of $bla_{CTX-M-1}$ group extended spectrum β-lactamase genes in *Escherichia coli* isolates from Tehran. Jundishapur Journal of Microbiology. 2013;**6**:e6863

[33] Ahmed MO, Clegg PD, Williams NJ, Baptiste KE, Bennett M. Antimicrobial resistance in equine faecal *Escherichia coli* isolates from North West England. Annals of Clinical Microbiology and Antimicrobials. 2010;**9**:12

[34] Luvsansharav UO, Hirai I, Niki M, Sasaki T, Makimoto K, Komalamisra C, et al. Analysis of risk factors for a high prevalence of extended-spectrum βlactamase-producing *Enterobacteriaceae* in asymptomatic individuals in rural Thailand. Journal of Medical Microbiology. 2011;**60**:619-624

[35] Li B, Sun JY, Liu QZ, Han LZ, Huang XH, Ni YX. High prevalence of CTX-M β-lactamases in faecal *Escherichia coli* strains from healthy humans in Fuzhou, China. Scandinavian Journal of Infectious Diseases. 2011;**43**:170-174

[36] Ahmed SF, Ali MMM, Mohamed ZK, Moussa TA, Klena JD. Fecal carriage of extended-spectrum β-lactamases and AmpC-producing *Escherichia coli* in a Libyan Community. Annals of Clinical Microbiology and Antimicrobials. 2014;**13**:22

[37] Dembélé R, Huovinen E, Yelbéogo D, Kuusi M, Sawadogo G, Haukka K, et al. Burden of acute gastrointestinal infections in Ouagadougou, Burkina Faso. Journal of Microbiology Infectious Diseases. 2016;**6**:45-52

[38] Rimal U, Thapa S, Maharajan R. Prevalence of extended spectrum beta-lactamase producing *Escherichia coli* and *Klebsiella* species from urinary specimens of children attending Friendship International Children's Hospital. Nepal Journal of Biotechnology. 2017;**5**:32-38

[39] Gupta V. An update on newer β-lactamases. The Indian Journal of Medical Research. 2007;**126**:417-427

[40] Sharma AR, Bhatta DR, Shrestha J, Banjara MR. Antimicrobial susceptibility pattern of *Escherichia coli* isolated from

urinary tract infected patients attending Bir Hospital. Nepal Journal of Science and Technology. 2013;**14**:177-184

[41] Monira S, Shabnam SA, Imran ASK, Sadique A, Johura FT, Rahman KZ, et al. Multi-drug resistant pathogenic bacteria in the gut of young children in Bangladesh. Gut Pathogenesis. 2017;**9**:19

[42] Abrar S, Ul AN, Liaqat H, Hussain S, Rasheed F, Riaz S. Distribution of *bla*CTX-M, *bla*TEM, *bla*SHV and *bla*OXA genes in extended-spectrum βlactamase-producing clinical isolates: A three-year multi-center study from Lahore, Pakistan. Antimicrobial Resistances and Infection Control. 2019;**8**:80

[43] Quan J, Zhao D, Liu L, Chen Y, Zhou J, Jiang Y, et al. High prevalence of ESBL producing *Escherichia coli* and *Klebsiella pneumoniae* in community-onset bloodstream infections in China. The Journal of Antimicrobial Chemotherapy. 2016;**72**(1):273-280

[44] Sonda T, Kumburu H, van Zwetselaar M, Alifrangis M, Mmbaga BT, Lund O, et al. Prevalence and risk factors for CTX-M gram-negative bacteria in hospitalized patients at a tertiary care hospital in Kilimanjaro, Tanzania. European Journal of Clinical Microbiology & Infectious Diseases. 2018;**37**:1-10

[45] Pavez M, Troncoso C, Osses I, Salazar R, Illesca V, Reydet P, et al. High prevalence of CTX-M-1 group in ESBL-producing *Enterobacteriaceae* infection in intensive care units in southern Chile. The Brazilian Journal of Infectious Diseases. 2019;**23**(2):102-110

[46] Ouchar Mahamat O, Tidjani A, Lounnas M, Hide M, Benavides J, Somasse C, et al. Fecal carriage of extended-spectrum βlactamase-producing *Enterobacteriaceae* in hospital and community settings in Chad. Antimicrobial Resistance and Infection Control. 2019;**8**:169

[47] Tani BA-KZ, Decré D, Genel N, Boucherit-Otmani Z, Arlet G, Drissi M. Molecular and epidemiological characterization of enterobacterial multidrug-resistant strains in Tlemcen Hospital (Algeria) (2008-2010). Microbial Drug Resistance. 2013;**19**(3):185-190

[48] Fashae K, Engelmann I, Monecke S, Braun DS, Ehricht R. Molecular characterisation of extended spectrum ß-lactamase producing *Escherichia coli* in wild birds and cattle, Ibadan, Nigeria. BMC Veterinary Research. 2021;**17**:33

[49] Gassama-Sow A, Aïdara-Kane A, Barraud O, Gatet M, Denis F, Ploy MC. High prevalence of trimethoprim-resistance cassettes in class 1 and 2 integrons in Senegalese *Shigella* spp isolates. Journal of Infection in Developing Countries. 2010;**4**:207-212

[50] Sambe-Ba B, Seck A, Wane AA, Fall-NiangNK,Gassama-SowA.Sensibilité aux antibiotiques et supports génétiques de la résistance des souches de *Shigella flexneri* isolées à Dakar de 2001 à 2010. Bulletin de la Societe de Pathologie Exotique. 2013;**106**:89-94

[51] Dembélé R, Kaboré WAD, Soulama I, Konaté A, Kagambèga A, Traoré O, et al. Involvement of class 1 and class 2 integrons in dissemination of *tet* and *cat*A1 resistance genes of *Salmonella enterica* from children with diarrhea in rural Burkina Faso. African Journal of Biotechnology. 2020b;**19**(1):1-7

[52] Bagré TS, Sambe-Ba B, Bawa-Ibrahim H, Bsadjo-Tchamba G, Dembélé R, Wane AA, et al. Isolation and characterization of enteropathogenic and enterotoxinogenic *Escherichia coli* from

dairy products consumed in Burkina Faso. African Journal of Microbiology Research. 2017;**11**(13):537-545

[53] Sáenz Y, Briñas L, Domínguez E, Ruiz J, Zarazaga M, Vila J, et al. Mechanisms of resistance in multiple-antibiotic-resistant *Escherichia coli* strains of human, animal, and food origins. Antimicrobial Agents and Chemotherapy. 2004;**48**:3996-4001

[54] Oliveira-Pinto C, Diamantino C, Oliveira PL, Reis MP, Costa PS, Paiva MC, et al. Occurrence and characterization of class 1 integrons in *Escherichia coli* from healthy individuals and those with urinary infection. Journal of Medical Microbiology. 2017;**66**(5):577-583

Chapter 9

Hidradenitis Suppurativa Perineal and Perianal

Rafael Luís Luporini, Sthefânia Mendonça Frizol, Maria Júlia Segantini, Leo Dantas Pereira, Alana Padilha Fontanella and Omar Féres

Abstract

Hidradenitis suppurativa (HS) is a chronic inflammatory, recurrent, and a debilitating skin disorder that affects the follicular epithelium, specifically of apocrine-gland-bearing regions (such as axillae, inframammary folds, groin, perineal, and/or perigenital). HS prevalence is around 1–4%, and the perineal disease is more common in males. HS is initially characterized by perifollicular lymphocytic infiltrate, which causes glands' duct occlusion, dilation, rupture of the follicle, and increased inflammation. The result is the formation of tunnels (fistulas) connecting the glands to the skin's surface. Secondary bacterial infections may occur. The etiological factors are obesity, smoking, and hormones, with a genetic predisposition of up to 40% of patients. HS usually occurs in early adulthood, with inflamed skin nodules, abscesses, pus discharge tunnels, and scarring developed in axillary, inguinal, gluteal, and perineal body sites. The diagnosis is made clinically based on typical lesions, affected regions, and progression (chronicity, persistent lesions, and recurrence). The therapy for HS must be individualized and guided by severity. They range from topical and systemic antibiotics, retinoids, immunosuppressive drugs, local therapies such as laser, phototherapy, hyperbaric, and even regulated and extensive surgical resections, which may be associated with skin grafts.

Keywords: hidradenitis suppurativa perineal, perianal diseases

1. Introduction

Hidradenitis suppurativa (HS) is characterized as a chronic inflammatory, recurrent, and debilitating skin disorder that affects the follicular epithelium, specifically of apocrine-gland-bearing regions such as axillae, inframammary folds, groin, perineal, and/or perigenital [1–3]. Even though HS is almost three times more common in women, the perineal disease is particularly seen more often in males, and it is related to higher morbidity compared to other regions [1, 2].

HS often presents with very painful, inflamed skin nodules, abscesses, pus-discharging tunnels (known as sinus tracts and fistulas), and scarring. The diagnosis is made clinically and based on typical lesions, affected regions, and progression (chronicity, persistent lesions, and recurrence) [3, 4]. HS is a difficult disease to diagnose, given its multiple differential diagnoses that can lead to erroneous conclusions, with a diagnostic delay that can reach 12 years, leading to disease recurrence and progression [1, 3, 4].

Owing to its diversified presentation, with intense chronic pain, continuous purulent secretion, and bad smell, HS has a profound negative influence on patients' private and professional lives, affecting their economic condition and quality of life. Thus, the topic deserves to be highlighted, since HS is a chronic disease with high morbidity and a negative impact on health systems and society [4].

2. Historical context

The term hidradenitis suppurativa is derived from the Greek words "*hidros*" (sweat) and "*aden*" (glands). Also known as reverse acne, it was first described by Velpeau, a French physician, in 1839, as superficial abscesses of a peculiar location, affecting the armpits, breasts, and perianal region [4, 5]. In 1854, the French surgeon Verneuil suggested some association based on clinical data with sweat glands and named the disease after him. In 1893, Pollitzer and Dubreuilh established a clear etiopathogenesis associated with apocrine sweat glands [5]. Despite these discoveries, there were not enough studies to understand HS as a disease until 1939, when Brunsting published a complete work on the subject [4–6].

3. Epidemiology

HS is a disease with few epidemiological data described in the literature, with a large part of North American and European studies. It was considered a rare condition, mainly due to diagnostic errors and underreporting existing cases [5, 7]. In young European population, its prevalence is around 1–4% globally [8, 9]. In the United States, a study in Minnesota estimated a prevalence value of 0.13%, which is lower than that presented in Europe [10]. Regarding the age group, the disease is common between puberty and 40 years of age, being more frequent between 21 and 29 years of age, tending to decrease and disappear in women after menopause [5, 7]. The occurrence in females is higher, with a ratio of three females to one male. Perineal and perianal disease is more prevalent in males and is also more severe and associated with an increased risk of degeneration to squamous cell carcinoma [7, 11]. A Dutch study shows that disease severity is closely linked to disease, body mass index, male gender, and smoking [12]. There is evidence that the higher the body mass index, the greater the severity of the disease. HS was 10 times more prevalent in the morbidly obese compared to the general population [12, 13]. The relationship between smoking and HS was related in 60–70% of patients, but not associated with disease severity. There is no pattern of racial or even ethnic predilection today [13, 14].

4. Etiology

Although the etiology of HS has not been fully elucidated, there is a genetic predisposition, as up to 40% of patients with HS have a positive family history. Some other factors not so well described may also be associated, such as hormonal changes and hyperandrogenic states, use of oral contraceptives, lithium, chemical irritants such as antiperspirants and deodorants, metabolic syndrome, inflammatory bowel disease, diabetes, and spondyloarthropathy that can lead to an increase in morbidity and mortality [15, 16].

Smoking and obesity are possible secondary causes of the disease and factors of worse prognosis. Some studies suggest that nicotine acts by stimulating and leading to dysfunctional glandular secretion, further altering neutrophil chemotaxis, leading to more severe diseases [13, 14]. Some studies have proven the association between smoking and perianal HS in 70% of patients; thus, one of the pillars of treatment is discouraging smoking [14–16].

Obesity can aggravate HS by retaining sweat and breaking the follicular and glandular ostia [15].

Bacterial colonization in HS is uncertain, being more associated as a secondary cause of the pathology. It can exacerbate the disease, but it is not a primary etiologic factor; there is no bacterial growth in more than half of the initial cases [15]. Bacterial infection occurs secondary to follicular occlusion. The most common bacteria are *Staphylococcus aureus* and *Staphylococcus epidermidis*. *Chlamydia trachomatis* and some anaerobes such as *Peptostreptococcus, Bacteroides,* and *Fusobacterium* can also be found. *Escherichia coli*, *Klebsiella*, and *Proteus* are more common in perineal HS [15, 16].

5. Pathogenesis

HS is initially characterized by perifollicular lymphocytic infiltrate, which causes glands' duct occlusion, dilation, and rupture of the follicle. The result is an increased inflammation that leads to the formation of tunnels connected to the surface of the skin and filled with debris (**Figure 1**) [14, 15].

Histologically, the skin is formed by three main layers: epidermis, dermis, and subcutaneous tissue. The invagination of the epidermis develops the skin appendages: hair follicles, apocrine glands, and eccrine glands. The sebaceous glands are located in the mid-dermis and are connected to the hair follicle. They can be unilobular or multilobular holocrine glands that secrete sebum to the skin surface. This oily substance is important to protect the skin from water loss and traumas and to provide antibacterial activity. Eccrine and apocrine glands are the two main types of human sweat glands. The eccrine glands have a straight eccrine duct and secretory coiled portion and are responsible for thermoregulation. The apocrine glands are larger and mainly located at the axillary and anogenital area, areolae, and eyelids [14, 15, 16].

These skin appendages are considered a peripheral endocrine organ, expressing receptors and synthesizing various hormones, especially the androgenic ones. During adolescence, the gonadal cells in the ovary and testis secrete estrogen and testosterone, leading to the development of secondary sexual characteristics, including pubic hairs and axillary hairs. In addition, the apocrine glands grow, and the sebum secretion increases. The body odor is mainly from the axillary apocrine sweat glands, related to the bacterial catabolism of apocrine sweat [14–16].

The HS affects these glands. Histopathological patterns of HS include hyperkeratosis of the terminal follicle openings, hyperplasia of follicular epithelium,

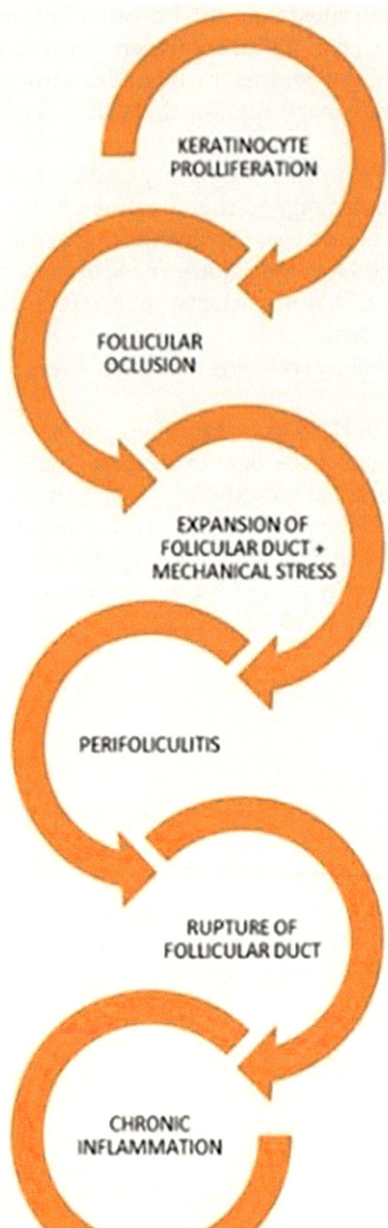

Figure 1.
Steps of hidradenitis suppurativa pathology.

and perifolliculitis. The disease is believed to begin with occlusion and dilation or elongation of the infundibular follicles. The infundibulum of the hair follicles then ruptures, followed by dermal suppurative inflammation with subsequent sinus tract formation and dermal fibrosis. This occlusion cause is not well understood.

The local microbiota may play a role in the innate immune system dysregulation [14, 17, 18].

The damaged skin in HS expresses more keratin 16 at the interfollicular epidermis and infundibulum. Therefore, it is believed that a genetic propensity must be related to the epidermal cell differentiation and innate immunity in HS, leading to ill skin. Infiltrating CD4 + T cells secreting interleukin 17 (IL-17) and interferon-gamma (IFN-γ) are increased in perilesional and lesional skin of patients with HS. In these cases, the keratinocytes also produce significantly more IL-6, IL-8, tumor necrosis factor-alpha (TNF-α), interferon-gamma-induced protein 10, and C-C motif chemokine ligand 5 [16–18].

There are also morphological changes of the apocrine glands in HS, but it is still controversial whether the apocrine glands initiate or participate in the development of HS. The apocrine glands are full of secretory cell-like materials [18, 19]. The basal membrane zone gets thick and inflamed, and secondary bacterial Zcolonization contributes to the diffuse dense inflammatory aggregated in the dermis with dilated vessels, fibrotic changes, and diminished or absent appendageal structures, including apocrine glands. Besides, the number of eccrine sweat glands is reduced, and the sebaceous glands have a smaller volume and less number of sebaceous glands in the axilla and/or groin. The effect of decreased sebaceous glands is a drop in antimicrobial peptides and impaired innate immunity. Expression of integrin α6β4 in sick sebaceous glands may be associated with a bacterial infection [17–19].

6. Differential diagnoses

The diagnosis of HS is delayed in most cases due to the numerous possible differential diagnoses, which generates a negative impact on the course of the disease. The differential diagnosis includes a range of possibilities such as anthrax, dermoid cyst, furunculosis, fistulas, abscesses, pilonidal cyst, cutaneous tuberculosis, and inflammatory bowel disease, among others shown in **Table 1** [20, 21].

The most important differential diagnosis of perianal and genital disease is subcutaneous tunneling diseases (e.g., pilonidal disease, Crohn' disease (CD), benign anal fistula, and granuloma inguinale). A biopsy may be performed to elucidate the case. What differentiates pilonidal disease from HS is the absence of midline pits over the

Differential diagnosis of hidradenitis suppurativa		
Noduloulcerative syphilis	Blastomycosis	Lymphogranuloma *venereum*
Cutaneous Crohn disease	Scrofuloderma – Tuberculosis	Donovanosis
Carbuncle	Neoplasms	Cutaneous actinomycosis
Epidermoid cyst	Erysipelas	Intergluteal pilonidal disease
Simple abscesses	Furuncle	Cat scratch disease

Adaptad from Zouboulis et al. [21].

Table 1.
Differential diagnosis of hidradenitis suppurativa.

sacrum. The absence of involvement of the anal canal distinguishes HS from CD and benign anal fistula. About 50% of CD patients develop perianal lesions very similar to HS [20–22].

7. Associated conditions

HS is a chronic inflammatory systemic disease. It may be associated with several other pathologies (**Table 2**) [21]. Metabolic syndrome affects at least 50% of patients with HS, with an increased cardiovascular risk [20, 23].

Some rheumatologic pathologies may also be related, such as pyogenic arthritis, spondyloarthritis, gangrenosum pyoderma, amyloidosis, and synovitis, acne, pustulosis, hyperostosis, and osteitis (SAPHO) syndrome [20–21].

Owing to chronic inflammation, patients with HS have an increased risk for malignancy, and squamous cell carcinoma is the worst complication [22].

Associated disease to hidradenitis suppurative
Follicular occlusive diseases
• Acnevulgaris
• Acne conglobate
• Dissecting cellulitis
• Intergluteal pilonidal diseases
Pigmentary disorders
• Dowling - Degos disease
• Kitamura disease
Rheumatologic diseases
• Arthritis
• Synovitis
• Amyloidosis
• SAPHO
Endocrinologic and hormonal diseases
• Grave's disease
• Hashimoto's thyroiditis
• Hyperandrogenism
Miscellaneous
• Fox-Fordyce disease
• Steatocystoma multiplex
• Pityriasis rubra pilaris
• Pyoderma gangrenosum
Adapted from Zouboulis et al. [21].

Table 2.
Associated disease to hidradenitis suppurativa.

Psychiatric pathologies, such as depression, panic syndrome, and suicidal ideation, are also reported [21, 23].

8. Diagnosis and classification

The absence of a pathognomonic test to identify HS may delay the diagnosis [21]. Three clinical diagnostic criteria are used: the presence of typical lesions, typically affected regions, and chronicity [24, 25].

The typical lesions are painful nodules, abscesses, suppurative sinus tracts, coalescing scars, and complex comedones. Pruritus, fetid smell, pain, and burning sensation are the most common symptoms. Affected regions must include at least one of the following: axillary, infra- and intermammary, inguinal, perineal, perianal, and gluteal regions. Chronicity is characterized by persisting lesions over 3 months or two recurrences within the period of 6 months. Secondary bacterial infection may also cause chronicity [21, 23–25].

Familiar HS history must be considered and a full skin examination performed to assess the severity and exclude other diagnoses [21, 26].

The skin biopsy may be useful and should be performed if there is suspicion of squamous cell carcinoma. A firm, nonfluctuant, nondraining, superficially eroded, or ulcerated mass are strong evidence of malignancy [22].

If there is a primary infectious disease or clinical evidence of secondary cellulitis, a culture may help [21, 25, 26].

High-frequency ultrasound and magnetic resonance are used to detect dermal and subcutaneous involvement, discriminating differential diagnosis, such as fistula [21, 27].

HS severity is classified by the Hurley classification, which defines three stages according to the number, chronicity, and coalescence of the lesions as shown in **Table 3** [21].

Sartorius scoring system and international hidradenitis suppurativa severity score system (IHS4), most appropriate to assess disease severity and grade of inflammation, was later proposed (**Tables 4** and **5**) [21, 24].

Three clinical subtypes of HS have been described: axillary-mammary, follicular, and gluteal. According to another classification by van der [26], there are six phenotypes of HS: (I) regular type; (II) frictional furuncle type; (III) scarring folliculitis type; (IV) conglobata type; (V) syndromic type; and (VI) ectopic type. Recently, it has been suggested to distinguish between a follicular subtype and an inflammatory phenotype, which is usually associated with a worse course of the disease [21, 26, 27].

Hurley staging—severity score	Clinical features
Stage I-Mild	Single or multiple abscesses without sinus tracts and scarring
Stage II-Moderate	Recurrent abscesses with sinus tracts and scarring
Stage III-Severe	Diffuse or multiple interconnected sinus tracts and abscesses across the entire area

Adaptad from Zouboulis et al. [21].

Table 3.
Hurley staging severity score.

Sartorious score
I—Anatomical region involved (axilla, groin, gluteal or other region or inframammary region left and/or right: 3 points per region).
II—Number and scores of lesions (abscesses, nodules, fistulas, scars: points per lesion of all regions involved: nodules 2, fistulas 4, scars 1, others 1).
III—The longest distance between two relevant lesions, i.e. nodules and fistulas, in each region, or size if only one lesion (<5 cm, 2 points; $<10cm$,4 points; $>10cm$,8 points).
IV—Are all lesions clearly separated by normal skin? In each region (yes 0 / no 6).
Adapted from Sartorius et al. [24].

Table 4.
Sartorious score.

International hidradenitis suppurativa severity score system (IHS4)
Number of nodules multiplied by 1
Number of abscesses multiplied by 2
Number of draining tunnels (fistulas/sinuses) multiplied by 4
A score of more than 3 = mild; 4-10 = moderate ;11 or more = severe
Adapted from Zouboulis et al. [21].

Table 5.
International Hidradenitis Suppurativa Severity Score System (IHS4).

9. Treatment

HS is a complex and difficult-to-treat disease, with success rates depending on the stage of the disease. To efficiently control it, a multidisciplinary treatment should be offered with an early approach, involving clinical and preventive measures, psychological support, and surgery [21, 28].

Behaviors to mitigate the disease development are smoking cessation, weight management, avoiding mechanical friction, chemical and physical irritants such as shaving, and the use of deodorants [17, 21].

Drug therapy ranges from topical and systemic antibiotics, anti-inflammatory agents, retinoids, antiandrogens, fumarates, and biguanides to immunosuppressive therapy. Local therapies, such as laser, phototherapy, hyperbaric, surgical resections, and skin grafts, can be useful [28, 29].

Topical antibiotics such as clindamycin were found to reduce nodules, pustules, and abscesses and should be used in mild-to-moderate disease with limited extent [21, 28]. On the other hand, systemic antibiotics are necessary in advanced disease commonly used for a long period (10–12 weeks). There is evidence supporting that the prescription of rifampicin and clindamycin soften the pain and lessen lesions count and suppuration [28]. In a randomized controlled trial, the combination of oral antibiotics (rifampicin and clindamycin) and 20 sessions of hyperbaric oxygen therapy was significantly superior to antibiotics alone in improving HS symptoms [29, 30].

Intralesional injections of glucocorticoids also play a role in the treatment of mild HS with few nodules and have shown to be effective and alleviate pain rapidly [21, 31].

Immunosuppressive drugs, such as tumor necrosis factor-alpha (TNF-α), interleukin-1 (IL-1), and interleukin-12/23 (IL-12/IL-23) inhibitors, are an option of treatment. Even though their effects were demonstrated mostly in small case series, there is strong evidence based on large randomized controlled trials supporting the use of adalimumab (anti-TNF). In one of these studies, patients received weekly dose of adalimumab and 58.9% of them achieved at least 50% of reduction in acute lesion count, with no increase in abscesses [31–33].

More effective treatment involves several therapeutic strategies together, considering the severity and distribution of the lesions. Clinical and social income conditions of the patient may be considered to guide the proper management [31–33].

Some studies indicated that the best perineal/perianal outcome with the lowest recurrence rate is the surgical removal of all apocrine tissue with ill glands and subsequent reconstruction [21, 28, 32].

Hidradenitis suppurativa treatment according to Hurley stage		
Adjuvant treatment (all stages)	• Weight loss and tobacco cessation • Pain control • Antimicrobial wash • Appropriate dressings • Psychosocial support measures • Management of concomitant comorbidities	
Hurley Stage 1 and II	Topical treatments	• Topical antibiotics and keratolytic agents (e.g. clindamycin lotion 1% bid for 3 months; resorcinol 15% bid) • Intralesional corticosteroids – triamcinolone
	Systemic treatments	• Oral antibiotics (e.g. oral tetracycline 500 mg bid for 4 month; dapsone 25-200 mg daily) • Systemic retinoids (e.g. acitretin 0.25 to 0.88 mg/kg daily; alitretinoin 10 mg daily) • Antiandrogenic therapies (e.g. oral contraceptive pills; finasteride 5 mg daily; metformin 500-1500 mg daily)
	Surgical/Physical Treatments	• Less invasive surgical approaches (e.g. local excision, curettage and electrocauterization, deroofing, punch debridement, cryoinsufflation) • Laser and lights therapy (e.g.Nd:YAG, CO2 laser, PUVA)
Hurley Stage II to III (includes Stage I to II approaches)	Systemic treatments	• Oral antibiotics (e.g. oral rifampin 600 mg daily + clindamycin 300 mg bid for 10 weeks) • Systemic immunosuppressants (e.g. ciclosporin 2-6 mg/kg/day) • Biological treatments (e.g. adalimumab 160 mg week 0,80 mg week 2 , then 40 mg weekly. Consider also, infliximab 5 mg/kg weeks 0,2 and 6; ustekinumab 45 or 90 mg at weeks 0,4,16 and 28)
	Surgical/Physical Treatments	• More invasive surgical approaches (e.g. wide radical excision)

Adapted from Zouboulis et al. [21], and Ingram et al. [28].
CO2: carbon dioxide; Nd:YAG: long-pulsed neodymium:yttrium-aluminum-garnet laser; IPL: intense pulse light; PDT: photodynamic therapy; and PUVA: bath psoralen plus ultraviolet A

Table 6.
Recommendations for surgical treatment of hidradenitis supurativa according to Hurley Stage.

As an adjuvant measure, the use of hyperbaric oxygen therapy has been satisfactory in cases of extensive surgical resections as well [29]. In addition, among patients undergoing postoperative reconstructions with the creation of flaps that evolve with complications, such as necrosis or infection, hyperbaric oxygen therapy presented excellent results, with a shorter healing time [28, 29, 33].

Treatment for HS is established according to the Hurley stage, which classifies it into three degrees of severity, as shown in **Table 6**.

Punch debridement is recommended to treat acute inflammatory nodes. This is known as the "mini unroofing" procedure: a single follicle is evacuated by partially removing its roof. Surgical unroofing (deroofing management) can also be performed in Hurley stages II or III [31, 33].

A similar procedure referred as skin-tissue-saving excision with electrosurgical peeling (STEEP) is an alternative to wide excision. It may be performed on local or extensively affected tissue areas. It consists of careful unroofing and debridement of sinuses and inflamed tissue followed by scrubbing. This can be alternatively made with a carbon dioxide laser [31–33].

Incision and drainage alone lead to high recurrence levels and are, therefore, not recommended as a single treatment. However, it may be useful for pain relief [33, 34].

Sweeping excision is used to manage an extensive area of chronic HS (Hurley stage III), particularly when conservative measures fail. It is not curative but generally leads to long periods without recurrence. The entire affected area is removed until the normal-appearing subcutaneous fat is evident [28, 34].

Figures 2–5 demonstrate selected cases of HS and extensive lesion resections.

In our experience, patients with mild/moderate HS confined to a small area tend to respond to clinical and simple pharmacological treatment (topical and/or oral antibiotics). In cases of refractoriness and high inflammatory activity, adalimumab associated with antibiotics should be a great option to control the symptoms and extension of HS.

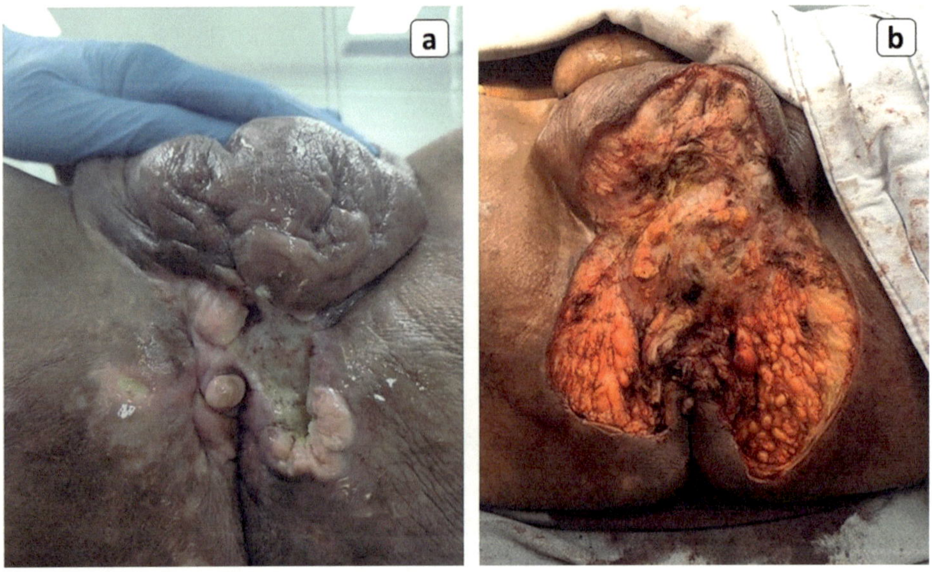

Figure 2.
Hidradenitis suppurativa lesions in the perianal and perineal region. (a) Preoperative and (b) immediate postoperative aspects.

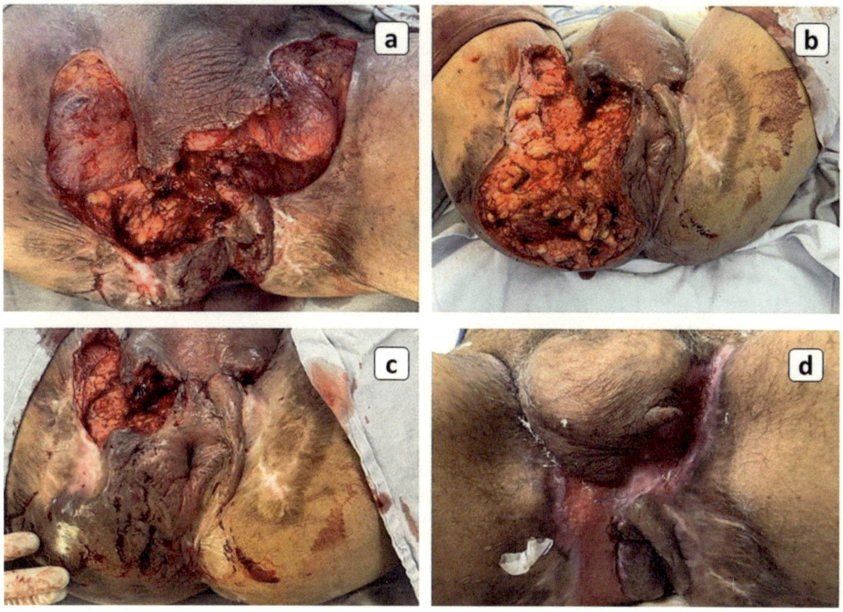

Figure 3.
Extensive HS resections (a, b, c—immediate and d—late).

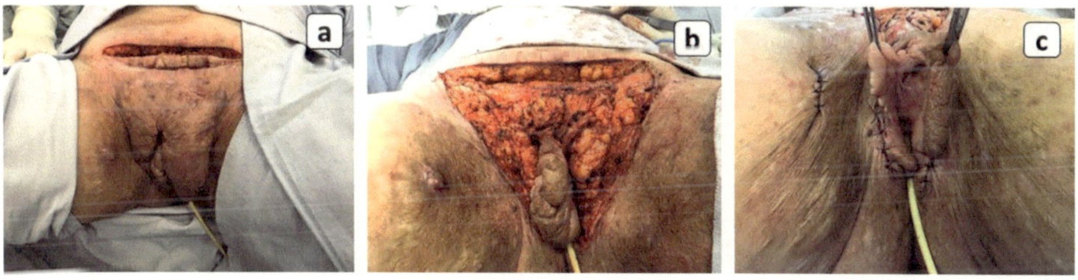

Figure 4.
Patient underwent modified radical vulvectomy. Preoperative (a), intraoperative (b), and reconstruction primary (c) image of the external genitalia marked scarring and fistulous tracts were evident in the pubis, vulva, and groin.

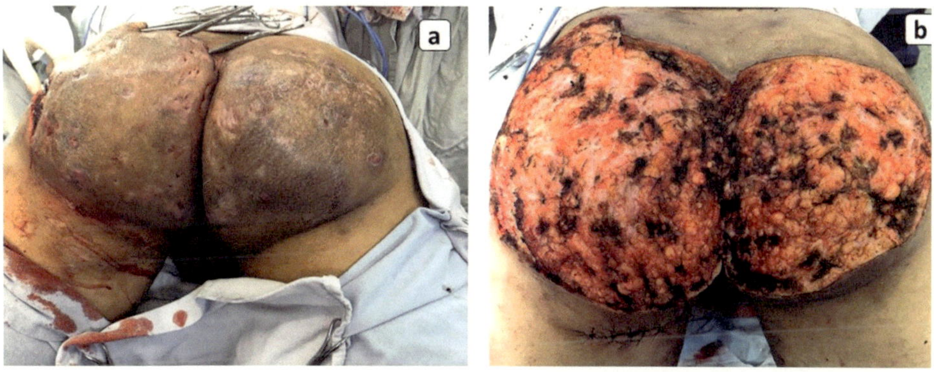

Figure 5.
Extensive resection in the gluteus and perineum of HS with closure by second intention. Preoperative (a) and postoperative (b) immediate.

Among patients presenting scars, tunnels, and contractures or chronic refractory lesions, surgery should be considered. Localized lesions allow small procedures such as deroofing; nevertheless, in severe and extensive injuries, the size of intervention associates inversely with recurrence rates.

10. Conclusions

HS is a chronic disease that causes significant weakness and suffering. Its onset in young adulthood leads to loss of productivity given the limiting nature of the disease. Treatment must be individualized, according to the extent, severity, and degree of interference in quality of life. Topical or oral antibiotic therapy may be effective to treat mild diseases in small areas. Biological agents can be applied to severe or widespread diseases. New treatment options are emerging to target inflammatory agents. Perianal, perineal, and refractory cases of HS should be vigorously treated. Best outcomes are achieved with large resections and reconstructive procedures.

Conflict of interest

The authors declare no conflict of interest.

Abbreviations

HS	hidradenitis suppurativa
CD	Crohn disease
IL	interleukin
TNF	tumor necrosis factor
SAPHO	pustulosis-hyperostosis syndrome
STEEP	skin-tissue-saving excision with electrosurgical peeling

Author details

Rafael Luís Luporini[1,2]*, Sthefânia Mendonça Frizol[2,3], Maria Júlia Segantini[3], Leo Dantas Pereira[3], Alana Padilha Fontanella[3] and Omar Féres[3]

1 Federal University of São Carlos, São Paulo, Brazil

2 Santa Casa de São Carlos, São Carlos, São Paulo, Brazil

3 Hospital das Clínicas de Ribeirão Preto – Universidade de São Paulo, São Paulo, Brazil

*Address all correspondence to: rafaelluporini@ufscar.br

References

[1] Seyed Jafari S, Hunger RE, Schlapbach C. Hidradenitis Suppurativa: Current understanding of pathogenic mechanisms and suggestion for treatment algorithm. Frontiers in Medicine. 2020;**7**(March):18-20. DOI: 10.3389/fmed.2020.00068

[2] Shah N. Hidradenitis suppurativa: A treatment challenge. American Family Physician. 2005;**72**(8):1547-1552

[3] Kagan RJ et al. Surgical treatment of hidradenitis suppurativa: A 10-year experience. Surgery. 2005;**138**(4):734-741

[4] Jemec GBE, Kimball AB. Hidradenitis suppurativa: Epidemiology and scope of the problem. Journal of the American Academy of Dermatology. 2015;**73**(5):S4-S7

[5] Barros DE, Resende MS, Macedo EJO, Araújo JJ, Mendes MB, Carvalho FA. Tratamento cirúrgico da hidradenite supurativa perianal. Rev bras Colo-Proct. 1988;**8**(3):98-101

[6] Golcman B, Tuma P Jr, Bonamichi GT, Faria JCM, Golcman R, Ferreira MC. Tratamento cirúrgico da hidradenite supurativa. Rev Hosp Clín Fac Med S Paulo. 1991;**46**(3):141-144

[7] Wang SC et al. Hidradenitis Suppurativa. Advances in Skin & Wound Care. 2015;**28**(7):325-332

[8] Revuz JE et al. Prevalence and factors associated with hidradenitis suppurativa: Results from two case-control studies. Journal of the American Academy of Dermatology. 2008;**59**(4):596-601

[9] Jemec G, Heidenheim M, Nielsen NH. The prevalence of hidradenitis suppurativa and its potential precursor lesions. Journal of the American Academy of Dermatology. 1996;**35**(2): 191-194

[10] Shahi V et al. Prevalence of Hidradenitis Suppurativa: A Population-Based Study in Olmsted County, Minnesota. Dermatology. 2014;**229**(2):154-158

[11] Chapman S, Delgadillo D, Barber C, Khachemoune A. Cutaneous squamous cell carcinoma complicating hidradenitis suppurativa: A review of the prevalence, pathogenesis, and treatment of this dreaded complication. Acta Dermatovenerologica Alpina Pannonica et Adriatica. 2018;**27**(1):25-28. DOI: 10.15570/actaapa.2018.5et

[12] Schrader AMR et al. Hidradenitis suppurativa: A retrospective study of 846 Dutch patients to identify factors associated with disease severity. Journal of the American Academy of Dermatology. 2014;**71**(3):460-467

[13] Kromann C et al. The influence of body weight on the prevalence and severity of Hidradenitis Suppurativa. Acta Dermato-Venereologica. 2014;**94**(5):553-557

[14] Acharya P, Mathur M. Hidradenitis suppurativa and smoking: A systematic review and meta-analysis. Journal of the American Academy of Dermatology. 2020;**82**(4):1006-1011

[15] Vinkel C, Thomsen SF. Hidradenitis Suppurativa: Causes, features, and current treatments. The Journal of Clinical and Aesthetic Dermatology. 2018;**11**(10):17-23

[16] Jemec GBE et al. The bacteriology of Hidradenitis suppurativa. Dermatology. 1996;**193**(3):203-206

[17] Hunger RE et al. Swiss practice recommendations for the management of

Hidradenitis Suppurativa/Acne Inversa. Dermatology. 2017;**233**(2-3):113-119

[18] Kurayev A, Ashkar H, Saraiya A, Gottlieb AB. Hidradenitis Suppurativa: Review of the pathogenesis and treatment. Journal of Drugs in Dermatology. 2016;**15**(8):1017-1022

[19] Prens E, Deckers I. Pathophysiology of hidradenitis suppurativa: An update. Journal of the American Academy of Dermatology. 2015;**73**(5):S8-S11

[20] Tsai S-J, Chu C-B, Yang C-C. Hidradenitis suppurativa: Disease pathophysiology and sex hormones. Chinese Journal of Physiology. 2021;**64**(6):257

[21] Zouboulis CC et al. European S1 guideline for the treatment of hidradenitis suppurativa/acne inversa. Journal of the European Academy of Dermatology and Venereology. 2015;**29**(4):619-644

[22] Jourabchi N et al. Squamous cell carcinoma complicating a chronic lesion of hidradenitis suppurativa: A case report and review of the literature. International Wound Journal. 2016;**14**(2):435-438

[23] Scala E et al. Hidradenitis Suppurativa: Where we are and where we are going. Cell. 2021;**10**(8):2094

[24] Sartorius K et al. Suggestions for uniform outcome variables when reporting treatment effects in hidradenitis suppurativa. British Journal of Dermatology. 2003;**149**(1):211-213

[25] Lowe MM, Naik HB, Clancy S, Pauli M, Smith KM, Bi Y, et al. Immunopathogenesis of hidradenitis suppurativa and response to anti-TNF-a therapy. JCI Insight, 2020;**5**:1-19. DOI: 10.1172/jci.insight.139932

[26] van der Zee HH, Jemec GB. New insights into the diagnosis of hidradenitis suppurativa: Clinical presentations and phenotypes. Journal of the American Academy of Dermatology. 2015 Nov;**73**(5 Suppl 1):S23-6. DOI: 10.1016/j.jaad.2015.07.047

[27] Jørgensen A-HR et al. Clinical, microbiological, immunological and imaging characteristics of tunnels and fistulas in hidradenitis suppurativa and Crohn's disease. Experimental Dermatology. 2019;**29**(2):118-123

[28] Ingram JR, Woo PN, Chua SL, Ormerod AD, Desai N, Kai AC, et al. Interventions for hidradenitis suppurativa: A Cochrane systematic review incorporating GRADE assessment of evidence quality. British Journal of Dermatology. 2016;**174**(5):970-978

[29] Ozdemir Y et al. Hyperbaric oxygen therapy for the management of postsurgical wounds in Hidradenitis Suppurativa. The American Surgeon. 2010;**76**(12):237-238

[30] Yildiz H et al. A prospective randomized controlled trial assessing the efficacy of adjunctive hyperbaric oxygen therapy in the treatment of hidradenitis suppurativa. International Journal of Dermatology. 2015;**55**(2):232-237

[31] Katzman JH, Tahmasbi M, Ghayouri M, Nanjappa S, Li MC, Greene J. Management of Severe Hidradenitis Suppurativa. Cureus, 2021;**13**(2):1-5. DOI: 10.7759/cureus.13483

[32] Duran C, Baumeister A. Recognition, diagnosis, and treatment of hidradenitis suppurativa. Journal of the American Academy of Physician Assistants. 2019;**32**(10):36-42

[33] Magalhães RF et al. Consensus on the treatment of hidradenitis suppurativa - Brazilian Society of Dermatology.

Anais Brasileiros de Dermatologia. 2019;**94**(2):7-19

[34] Formiga GJS, Horta SHC, Boratto SF, Silva JH. Hidradenite supurativa perineal. Avaliação do tratamento cirúrgico em 18 anos de experiência GALDINO. Rev bras Colo-Proct. 1997;**17**(2):101-104

Chapter 10

Perspective Chapter: Management of Pruritus Ani

Nathalie Mantilla and Juaquito Jorge

Abstract

Pruritus ani is a benign anorectal disorder characterized by an itching sensation of the perianal skin. It is a source of embarrassment and frustration for those who suffer from it. Multiple conditions can be responsible for perianal itching; however, most cases are idiopathic. Skin breakdown from constant scratching creates a vicious cycle exacerbating the symptoms. Empiric treatment resolves the problem in most cases, but additional testing should be performed when deemed necessary. Guided management to control associated diseases, lifestyle modifications, as well as skin protection, is paramount in the management.

Keywords: pruritus, itching, perianal skin, irritation

1. Introduction

Anal pruritus is an uncomfortable condition that often isolates patients and causes delays in seeking medical attention due to embarrassment. Pruritus ani is a benign condition defined as itching or burning sensation of the skin of the perianal region [1]. In many cases, multiple factors are implicated, making a precise diagnosis challenging. Typically, patients present after attempting home remedies and over-the-counter medications, compounded by embarrassment to discuss these symptoms with healthcare professionals. Undoubtedly, pruritus ani is an unpleasant sensation that can greatly impact the quality of life of affected patients. The incidence in the general population is estimated to be up to 5%, affecting men in a greater proportion compared with women (4:1 ratio). Commonly, diagnosis is made in the fourth to sixth decades of life, with a slow progression of symptoms that worsen particularly at night and in warm weather due to excessive moisture of the perianal area [2–4].

Depending on the degree of involvement of the perianal skin, pruritus ani can be localized or diffuse and classified into primary (idiopathic) or secondary (associated with other pathologies) [5]. Multiple conditions have been implicated in the etiology of pruritus ani, perianal eczema being the most common cause.

2. Pathophysiology and etiology

The differential diagnosis of pruritus ani comprises a long list of conditions that can be grouped into infectious, inflammatory, and neoplastic. Primary or idiopathic pruritus ani accounts for more than half of cases (50–90%), and a variety of factors have been implicated in the pathophysiology (anatomic, dietary, hygienic, psychogenic, local irritants, and medications) [6]. However, fecal contamination and local skin irritation are the most common provoking factors. This phenomenon occurs by the activation of non-myelinated C-fibers in the epidermis and sub-dermis; though, the neurophysiological mechanisms behind the symptoms are much more complex. Scratching, although temporarily alleviates the itching sensation, is thought to produce inadequate feedback to inhibit further symptoms (*puritoceptive itching*). Therefore, avoiding scratching is key in the interruption of the vicious cycle of skin trauma, which is an additional stimulus for itching. In our practice, as part of routine interrogation and physical examination, we always inquire about products patients may have applied for symptomatic relief. Despite most patients denying fecal incontinence, many have some degree of leakage demonstrated during the examination of the perianal area and confirming the presence of stool.

Infectious
Bacterial
Fungal
Viral
Parasitic
Dermatologic
Psoriasis
Lichen planus, lichen simplex chronicus, lichen sclerosus
Contact dermatitis
Atopic dermatitis
Perianal psoriasis
Systemic diseases
Diabetes mellitus
Leukemia, lymphoma, polycythemia vera
Liver disease (hyperbillirubinemia)
Chronic renal failure
Thyroid disorders (hyperthyroidism)
Anorectal diseases
Benign
Hemorrhoids (internal and external)
Rectal prolapse (mucosal and full thickness)
Fissure
Fistula-in-ano
Diarrhea
Secreting villous tumors
Fecal soiling and incontinence
Skin tags
Perianal Crohn's disease
Hidradenitis suppurativa
Malignant
Anal canal and anal margin cancer
Rectal cancer
Bowen's disease
Perianal Paget's disease
Miscellaneous
Radiation-induced dermatitis
Vaginal discharge
Urinary incontinence

Table 1.
Secondary pruritus—causes.

Several foods have been associated with the production of perianal itching and are commonly excluded from the diet as part of the initial management. These *pruritogenic foods* include coffee, colas, citrus fruits, chocolate, tea, energy drinks, alcoholic beverages, tomato, and spicy foods. They act as irritants of the perianal skin and have also been implicated in altering bowel habits, stool consistency, and facilitating seepage. A comprehensive history and physical examination are critical in narrowing the diagnosis since in many cases both primary and secondary etiologies can be found.

Secondary pruritus should be considered in cases where an identifiable cause is found. The etiologies in this group are very broad and can be classified into five categories—infectious, dermatologic, systemic disease, benign and malignant anorectal diseases, and miscellaneous (**Table 1**) [2, 3].

2.1 Infectious

Among the infectious agents, sexually transmitted diseases are common causes of anal pruritus, particularly in patients practicing anoreceptive intercourse. The most common pathogens are *Neisseria gonorrhoeae*, *Chlamydia trachomatis*, and *Treponema pallidum*, but herpes infections, molluscum contagiosum, and condyloma acuminatum (human papillomavirus infection) are also encountered (**Figure 1**). Herpetic lesions are typically painful vesicles with associated perianal burning sensation, that after rupture can leave superficial skin ulcerations (**Figure 2**). We often receive referrals of patients with a history of anoreceptive intercourse, as well as a large population of Human Immunodeficiency Virus (HIV) positive patients with perianal irritation. In most of these cases, symptoms are caused by undiagnosed sexually transmitted diseases (STD). Symptoms usually resolve after appropriate treatment.

In children, it has been well reported that *Beta-hemolytic streptococci* are involved in many cases of perianal dermatitis, whereas *Staphylococcus aureus* is frequently implicated in refractory dermatitis in adults. *Corynebacterium minutissimum* is the causative agent of erythrasma, a superficial infection of the intertriginous skin often seen in warm weather [7]. Fungal infections account for 10–43% of secondary anal pruritus, with *Candida albicans* being the most common fungi identified [8]. Parasitic perianal infections are rare, but common parasites identified include *Enterobius vermicularis* (pinworms), *Sarcoptes scabiei* (scabies), and pediculosis pubis [2]. Nocturnal and post-defecation pruritus ani in children is a characteristic symptom of pinworms infection. We do not have experience with pruritus ani in children since our practice is limited to adults only.

2.2 Dermatologic

A wide variety of dermatologic conditions have been associated with pruritus ani; hence, a detailed history and physical examination are essential. Perianal eczema is the most common condition responsible for anal pruritus. It originates as contact dermatitis to certain hygiene products or medications used to treat other anorectal conditions, such as over-the-counter hemorrhoid ointments, deodorants, scented wipes or toilet paper, and soaps. Inquiry about anal hygiene habits and products used must be part of the history. These patients often have a history of other atopic conditions, such as asthma. We typically encounter patients presenting with eczema after weeks of using over-the-counter products, such as moist wipes, and ointments to treat hemorrhoids.

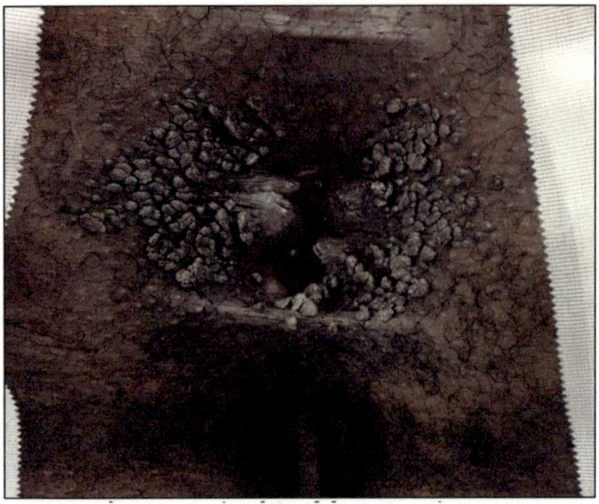

Figure 1.
Perianal condyloma acuminatum.

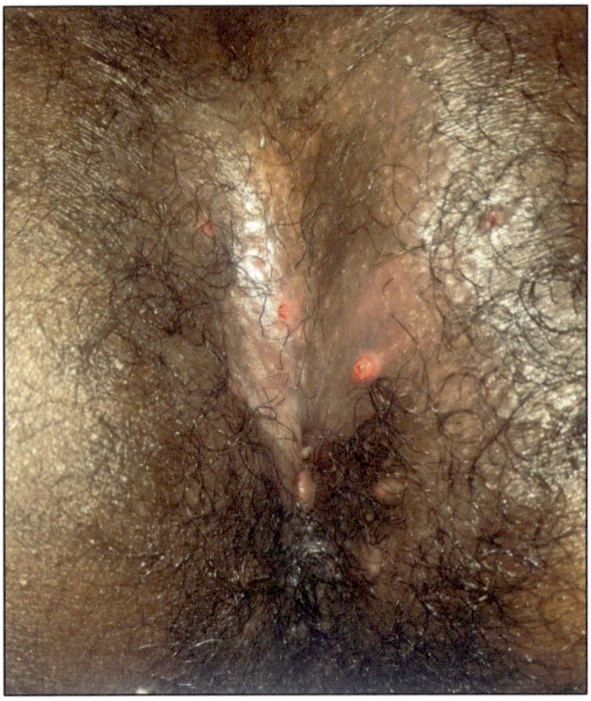

Figure 2.
Perianal herpes virus infection.

Atopic dermatitis is another common cause of pruritus ani, with an estimated frequency of 15–20% of the population [8]. Psoriasis is another skin problem associated with perianal pruritus, and although not as common, reports in the literature vary from 5 to 50% [8, 9]. Other less common dermatologic conditions that cause pruritus ani include seborrheic dermatitis, lichen planus, lichen sclerosus, and lichen simplex chronicus. A high index of suspicion is necessary for an adequate diagnosis and treatment.

2.3 Systemic diseases

Multiple systemic diseases have been associated with pruritus ani. While the underline triggering mechanisms are not known, treating the primary problem appears to alleviate the symptoms. Diabetes mellitus is one of the common diseases associated with anal pruritus, followed by liver disease (cholestasis), leukemia, lymphoma, chronic renal failure (uremic pruritus), pellagra, iron deficiency anemia, vitamin A and D deficiency, and hyperthyroidism [2, 3, 8].

2.4 Anorectal diseases

Pruritus ani is commonly found in patients with numerous benign anorectal conditions, such as external and internal hemorrhoids (**Figure 3**), anal fissures and fistulas (**Figure 4**), hidradenitis suppurativa, perianal Crohn's disease, anal skin tags, and pilonidal disease. Symptoms can be caused by the disease itself, as well as from local skin irritation associated with fecal soiling, prolapsing tissue, mucus discharge, chronic drainage, etc. Perianal diseases commonly interfere with local hygiene, leading to skin irritation from residual fecal material. Management of the perianal condition is necessary and may improve symptoms, as it has been seen in patients with prolapsing hemorrhoids after hemorrhoidectomy [10]. One of the most common situations we encounter in our clinic are patients confusing pruritus ani with symptomatic hemorrhoids, driving many to self-medicate and worsen symptoms.

Malignant anorectal processes can also provoke pruritus ani and should be considered and ruled out when appropriate. Among these, diseases are anal canal

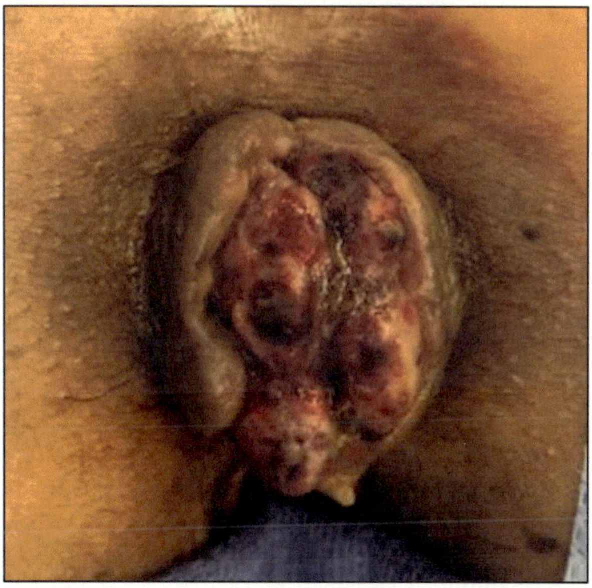

Figure 3.
Prolapse internal hemorrhoids. Courtesy of Arcila E, MD. Chicago, IL.

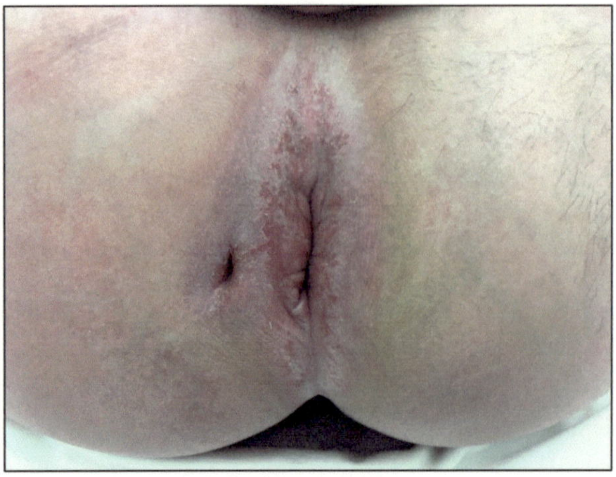

Figure 4.
Anorectal fistula with perianal dermatitis due to chronic drainage. Courtesy of Young D, MD. Chicago, IL.

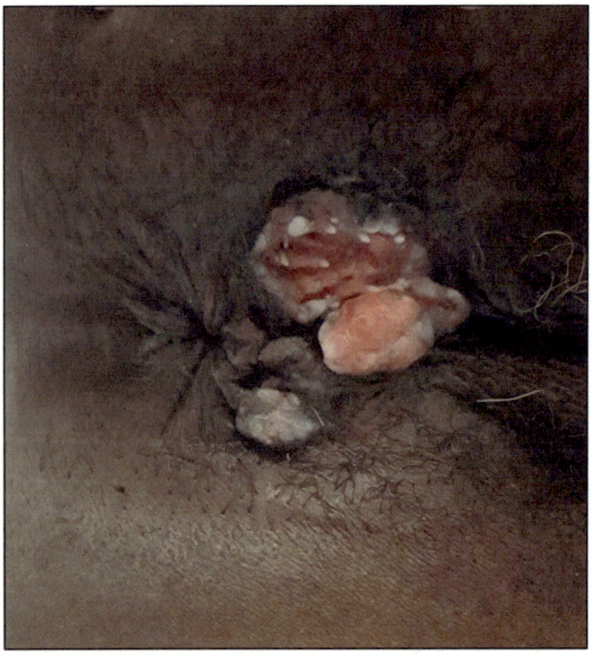

Figure 5.
Squamous cell carcinoma of the anal margin.

and anal margin cancer (**Figure 5**), low rectal cancer, Bowen's disease, or perianal squamous cell carcinoma *in situ* (**Figure 6**), and Paget's disease or cutaneous adenocarcinoma *in situ*. In patients with premalignant perianal lesions, such as anal intraepithelial neoplasia (AIN) caused by human papillomavirus infection (HPV), pruritus ani can be caused by the anal condyloma itself rather than the presence of dysplasia. The most common extra-mammary area affected by Paget's disease is the perianal region, occurring more frequently in white women in the sixth decade of life. In these cases, further evaluation of the gastrointestinal, urinary, and

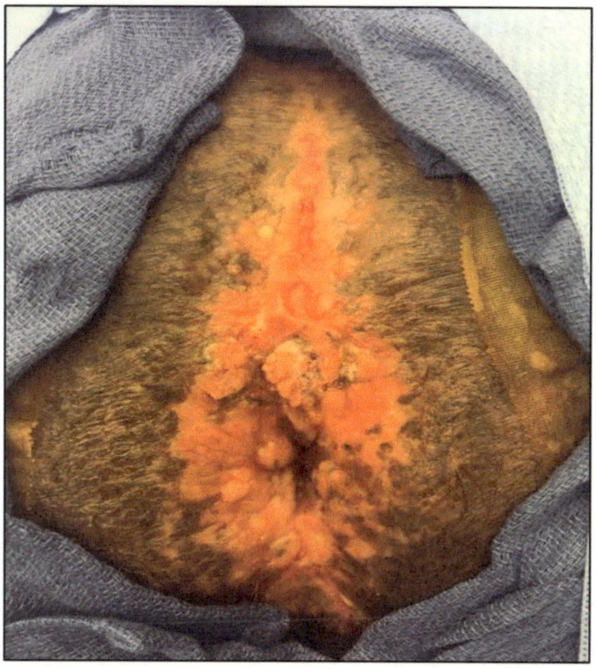

Figure 6.
Bowen's disease.

gynecologic systems is warranted, attributable to the high incidence of associated malignancy (33–86%) [11, 12].

2.5 Miscellaneous

Radiation-induced perianal dermatitis is an undesired side effect of cancer treatments. Multiple grading systems have been used to grade skin damage from radiation [13]. Regardless of the stage of dermatitis, from dry desquamation to breakdown and ulceration of the skin, many patients experience anal pruritus. Excessive moisture of the perianal skin from urinary incontinence or vaginal discharge is also associated with skin irritation and consequent pruritus ani. One of our hospitals is a high-volume center for the management of rectal and anal cancer. We often treat patients with sequelae of pelvic radiation, with fecal incontinence, perianal irritation, and consequent pruritus among the most common.

3. Evaluation and diagnosis

3.1 Clinical history

Patients with pruritus ani are often seen by a specialist after other treatments have failed, creating a challenge to establish a precise diagnosis. Clinical information, including presenting and associated symptoms, disease progression, co-morbidities, allergies, and medications, is warranted. Specifics about diet, sexual conduct, bowel habits, hygiene products and behaviors, and prior use of local agents should be part of the initial clinical encounter. History of atopia, anorectal disorders or surgeries, sexually transmitted

	Physical findings
Stage 0	Normal-appearing perianal skin
Stage I	Erythematous and inflamed perianal skin
Stage II	White, lichenified perianal skin
Stage III	Lichenified skin with coarse ridges and ulceration

Table 2.
The Washington hospital staging criteria.

diseases, among others, can aid in narrowing the differential diagnoses. During the initial interview, we focus on any potential triggers associated with the beginning of symptoms, instead of recent treatments that may have changed the course of the disease.

3.2 Physical examination

Inspection of the perianal area, perineum, and genitalia should be the first step of the physical examination. The examiner should look for erythema, blisters, ulcerations, maceration of the skin, residual fecal material, drainage, scratch marks, etc. If creams or ointments have been applied, they must be gently cleansed to expose the area for proper evaluation. In the early stages of the disease, no obvious abnormalities are found on the initial evaluation. A digital anorectal exam followed by a circumferential anoscopy should be performed to rule out anal canal conditions, however, any painful maneuvers should be avoided and, in most cases, these procedures are deferred until some of the pain and discomfort have subsided.

The Washington criteria, developed at the Washington Hospital Center, are commonly used to classify the severity of the pruritus ani based on clinical findings (**Table 2**) [8, 14]. In patients with Stage I disease, erythematous inflamed skin may be the only finding. In Stage II, there is lichenified perianal skin because of excessive itching and scratching or rubbing of the skin, resulting in thick leathery appearing skin. In addition to these changes, Stage III patients exhibit the presence of coarse ridges and ulceration of the affected skin. These staging criteria should be documented during clinic encounters, as it is useful for follow-up and evaluation of the response to treatment.

Microbiology testing should be performed based on the index of suspicion and clinical findings. To avoid misleading results, appropriate sample collection and specimens' manipulation is essential. For example, when feasible, drainage, or secretions should be aspirated with a syringe and placed in a sterile container, viral cultures should be kept on ice for transportation, etc. In patients with diarrhea, bacterial stool cultures, as well as ova and parasites testing, must be included.

When considered appropriate, a more extensive endoscopic examination can be performed, including examination under anesthesia, flexible sigmoidoscopy, and colonoscopy with tissue sampling for biopsies and cultures. With non-healing skin lesions that persist despite appropriate treatment, a biopsy to rule out malignancy is indicated.

4. Management

The initial goal of management of patients with pruritus ani should be directed to the relief of symptoms, healing of impaired skin, and protection and prevention of additional damage. In cases where a causative agent is identified (e.g., allergen and local irritant), further contact with the perianal skin must be avoided. Ultimately, treatment of underlying conditions in cases of secondary pruritus should lead to improvement of symptoms.

4.1 Education and lifestyle modifications

Particularly important in the management of idiopathic pruritus, a set of general strategies and recommendations should be implemented on the initial consultation. These changes are intended to restore the integrity of the perianal skin and prevent further damage when there is no underlying condition responsible for the symptoms. Patients should be instructed to avoid applying any home remedies, over-the-counter products, perfumed wipes, powders, lotions, soaps, etc. Education about gentle cleaning of the perianal area is also important, using water and unscented hypoallergenic soaps, followed by cool air-drying the area or by dabbing with toilet paper. We emphasize the importance of only applying creams and ointments prescribed by one member of our team. A proper balance between dryness and moist of the perianal area is vital. This can be achieved by placing a cotton ball or a makeup removal pad after cleaning, which will aid to keep the moisture of the zone balanced. Patients should also avoid tight-fitting underclothing and synthetic fabrics, especially in warm climates. Maintaining regular bowel habits is very important and controlling stool consistency may reduce the chances of stool leakage and soiling [8]. As part of the initial treatment, we regularly include a standard bowel regimen containing bulking agents, such as fiber supplements (usually powders to be dissolved in water) and stool softener when appropriate. Dietary recommendations for patients affected by pruritus ani have significant value; the elimination of the *pruritogenic foods* from the diet has shown significant improvement of symptoms in up to 48% of patients after 2 weeks (**Table 3**) [8, 15]. We routinely provide patients with a similar list of foods that can trigger or worsen symptoms and instruct them to avoid those at least for the first few weeks.

4.2 Topical agents

If there is persistent symptomatology after 2 weeks of uninterrupted proper treatment, special attention should be placed on excluding other etiologies of secondary

Caffeine-containing products
Colas
Coffee
Tea
Energy drinks
Citrus fruits and vegetables
Carbonated beverages
Chocolate
Tomato
Beer
Spicy and acidic foods
Refined carbohydrates
Nuts

Table 3.
Food products that contribute to pruritus ani symptoms.

pruritus. Only after infectious causes have been eliminated from the differential diagnosis, should topical steroids be considered for a limited time. Low-potency topical steroids such as hydrocortisone 1% are preferred as first-line treatment and have shown good results, by decreasing symptoms rapidly and consequently improving the quality of life [15]. The duration of therapy should not exceed 8 weeks since prolonged therapy or the use of potent steroids can be rather detrimental by causing skin atrophy and worsening of anal pruritus. Substance P is a neuropeptide that triggers itching and burning pain; Capsaicin decreases its levels, successfully treating the symptoms in up to 70% of patients when compared to placebo [16]. Topical steroids and capsaicin should be applied over clean and dry perianal skin in the morning and at night. After completion of therapy, this topical preparation should be replaced by a zinc oxide-based skin protectant, such as Calmoseptin® (Calmoseptine, Inc., Huntington Beach, CA). In our practice, we have noticed quick resolution of symptoms by applying vitamin petrolatum and lanolin-based ointments, such as those used in babies' diaper rash (A&D®, Bayer).

In rare cases of idiopathic pruritus ani, symptoms may persist and become intractable, despite all adequate treatment strategies, and after possible secondary causes have been excluded. Fortunately, for this small subset of patients, intradermal injection of methylene blue has been described with acceptable success [7, 8, 17]. Destruction of nerve terminations in the perianal area responsible for the symptoms is assumed as the mechanism of symptomatic relief. The technique description, including concentration and combination of drugs, varies slightly among reports. Full-thickness skin necrosis is a reported complication of this treatment [17, 18]. Our scant experience with this type of treatment has shown good results, however, when we need to use it, it is usually as a last resort.

5. Summary

Pruritus ani is a common benign anorectal condition that can be debilitating and frustrating for patients who suffer from it. A detailed clinical history and physical examination are of utmost importance to establish a diagnosis. When secondary pruritus is identified, the treatment should be tailored to the underlying condition. Biopsies, cultures, and other special testing methods should be performed when considered appropriate. Most of the cases improve with education and lifestyle modifications, such as cleansing habits and removing offending agents.

Author details

Nathalie Mantilla[1,2*] and Juaquito Jorge[3,4]

1 John H. Stroger Jr. Hospital of Cook County, Chicago, IL, United States

2 Rush University, Chicago, IL, United States

3 Tiesenga Surgical Associates, Elmwood Park, IL, United States

4 West Suburban Medical Center, Oak Park, IL, United States

*Address all correspondence to: nathaliemantilla@gmail.com

References

[1] Billingham RP, Isler JT, Kimmins MH, et al. The diagnosis and management of common anorectal disorders. Current Problems in Surgery. 2004;**33**(7):586-645

[2] Hanno R, Murphy P. Pruritus ani: Classification and management. Dermatologic Clinics. 1987;**5**(4):811-816

[3] Zuccati G, Lotti T, Mastrolorenzo A, et al. Pruritus ani. Dermatologic Therapy. 2005;**18**(4):355-362

[4] Mazier WP. Hemorrhoids, fissures, and pruritus ani. The Surgical Clinics of North America. 1994;**74**(6):1277-1292

[5] Metcalf A. Anorectal disorders. Five common causes of pain, itching and bleeding. Postgraduate Medicine. 1995;**98**(5):81-4, 87-9, 92-4

[6] Stamos MJ, Hicks TC. Pruritus ani: Diagnosis and treatment. Perspectives in Colon and Rectal Surgery. 1998; **11**(1):1-20

[7] Siddiqi S, Vijay V, Ward M, et al. Pruritus ani. Annals of the Royal College of Surgeons of England. 2008;**90**(6):457-463

[8] Steele SR et al. The ASCRS textbook of colon and rectal surgery. In: Gaertner WB, Melton GB, editors. Dermatology and Pruritus Ani. Third ed. Cham, Arlington Heights, IL, USA: Springer, The American Society of Colon and Rectal Surgeons; 2016. pp. 309-324

[9] Smith LE, Henrichs D, McCullah RD. Prospective studies on the etiology and treatment of pruritus ani. Diseases of the Colon and Rectum. 1982;**25**:358-363

[10] Murie JA, Sim AJ, Mackenzie I. The importance of pain, pruritus and soiling as symptoms of haemorrhoids and their response to haemorrhoidectomy or rubber band ligation. The British Journal of Surgery. 1981;**68**:247-249

[11] Perez DR, Trakarnsanga A, Shia J, Nash GM, Temple LK, Paty PB, et al. Management and outcome of perianal Paget's disease: A 6-decade institutional experience. Diseases of the Colon and Rectum. 2014;**57**(6):747-751

[12] Sarmiento JM, Wolff BG, Burgart LJ, Frizelle FA, Ilstrup DM. Paget's disease of the perianal region—An aggressive disease? Diseases of the Colon and Rectum. 1997;**40**:1187-1194

[13] Leventhal J, Young MR. Radiation dermatitis: Recognition, prevention, and management. Oncology (Williston Park, N.Y.). 2017;**31**(12):885-7, 894-9

[14] Gordon PH, Nivatvongs S. Perianal dermatologic disease. In: Gordon PH, editor. Principles and Practice of Surgery for the colon, Rectum and Anus. 3rd ed. New York, NY: Informa Healthcare; 2007. pp. 247-273

[15] Al-Ghnaniem R, Short K, Pullen A, et al. 1% hydrocortisone ointment is an effective treatment of pruritus ani: A pilot randomized controlled crossover trial. International Journal of Colorectal Disease. 2007;**22**(12):1463-1467

[16] Lysy J, Sistiery-Ittah M, Israelit Y, et al. Topical capsaicin—A novel and effective treatment for idiopathic intractable pruritus ani: A randomized, placebo controlled, crossover study. Gut. 2003;**52**(9):1323-1326

[17] Eusebio EB, Graham J, Mody N. Treatment of intractable pruritus ani.

Diseases of the Colon and Rectum. 1990;**33**(9):770-772

[18] Mentes BB, Akin M, Leventoglu S, et al. Intradermal methylene blue injection for the treatment of intractable idiopathic pruritus ani: Results of 30 cases. Techniques in Coloproctology. 2004;**8**(1):11-14

Chapter 11

Diarrhea: Novel Advances and Future Perspectives in the Etiological Diagnosis and Management

Zeeshan Javed, Muhammad Asrar, Bilal Rasool, Rabia Batool, Muhammad Asad Mangat, Usama Saleem, Muhammad Imran and Amna Batool

Abstract

Diarrhea is an increase in the incidence and fluidity of feces that is greatest characterized by duration (acute versus chronic), pathophysiologic apparatus, and anatomic location. Different types of diarrhea influence the health of both sexes. Infectious diarrhea is a big issue in many underdeveloped nations, with a high death rate, specifically among children under the age of five. Water diarrhea can be caused by a variety of microorganisms, including viruses, bacteria, and parasites. Acute bloody diarrhea is a health emergency that should be treated quickly. Most instances of acute diarrhea are clear on their own days without remedy. If you have adopted lifestyle adjustments and domestic remedies for diarrhea without achievement, there these are thought to be clinical remedies. By proper sanitation, hygiene protection, hand washing, food hygiene, and vaccination are required to control diarrhea.

Keywords: fluidity, infectious, remedies, instance, incidence, sanitation

1. Introduction

Higher cases of diarrhea are seen in developing countries. In which 14% of children aged fewer than five years had diarrhea, reported in a health survey of Nepal Demographic 2011. During the last three years, diarrhea cases in Nepal were increasing with time. It is estimated that out of 1000 children, 528–629 children are affected by it. During 2013–2014, in Nepal, 36 children per 1000 under less than five years of age die due to this infection [1]. In 2015, 9% of children less than five years of age are affected by diarrhea worldwide 1400 children are died due to it each day and annually 530,000 children are died due to it. Death rates of diarrhea are high in less than two years of children in Asia and Africa [2].

In Ethiopia, it is a very serious health problem for children in the region. In 2011, 13% of Children, less than five years of age were affected by this disease [3] 24–30% of the infant died due to diarrhea in this country [4]. The Ethiopian region is the very poorest region in the world and shows a high mortality rate of diarrhea [5] 15% of children having an age of fewer than five years are died due to it in developing countries. Acute diarrhea is a major cause of health problems worldwide. In 1973, rotavirus was the first time introduced as the cause of diarrhea when it was collected from epithelium cells of the upper villi surface in the gastrointestinal tract. Rotavirus was first seen in electro micrograph in 1973 and the word rotavirus has an origin from the Latin word, which means wheel-like. At the end of 1973, many types of research were conducted by doctors to determine the virus that caused diarrhea in infants and young children [6].

In the same year, the first-time rotavirus was identified in humans, when the first child is admitted to the hospital due to acute diarrhea. It was present in the cytoplasm of duodenal epithelial cells [7]. In Pakistan every year one child dies due to diarrhea. 400,000 infants die in his/her first years of life, published in the annual report in 2011 of Pakistan Medical Association. Acute diarrhea is a major problem in most developing countries. Most children remain under the threat of acute diarrhea infection during the first five years of life. It is estimated that 4.6 million deaths of children occurred annually in which acute diarrhea is the main factor of 25–30% of death of children aged less than five years [8]. 1.7 million children are infected by diarrhea worldwide, according to the world health organization. 760,000 mortalities of children occur each year due to diarrhea, which is why it is considered as the second major cause of death in children aged less than five years [9, 10].

2. Definition

Diarrhea is an increase in the incidence and fluidity of feces that is greatest characterized by duration (acute versus chronic), pathophysiologic apparatus, and anatomic location or the way of three or more loose or liquid couches per day it may also be described as a more common passage than is the normal for the individual.

3. Types of diarrhea

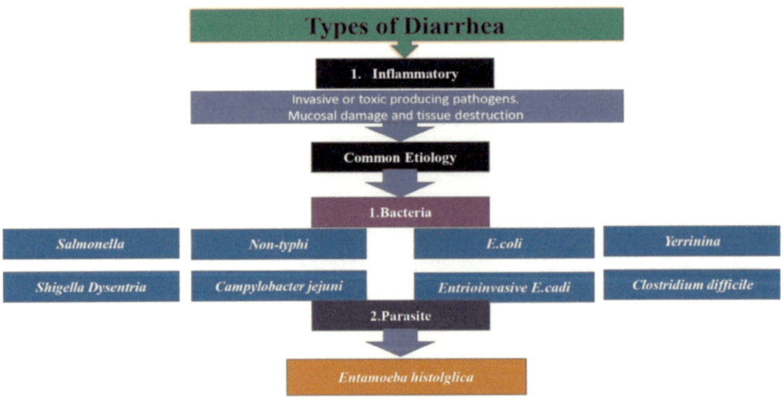

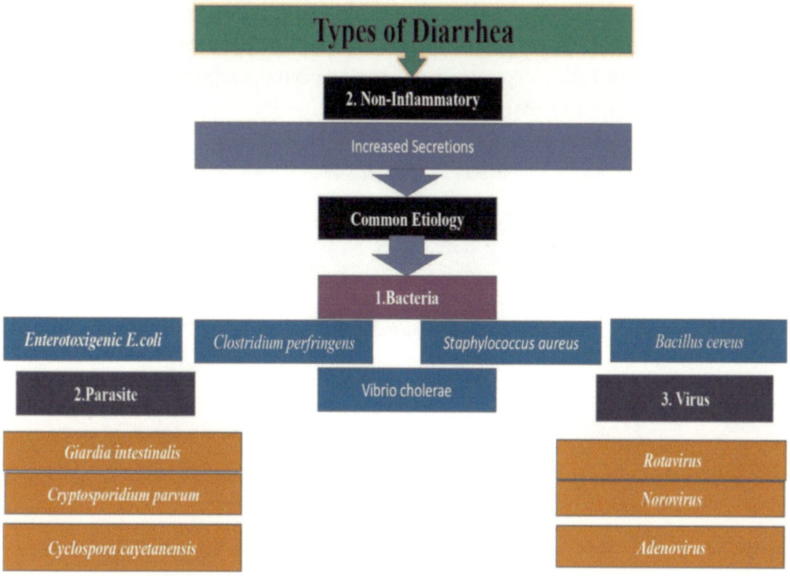

3.1 Acute watery diarrhea

It lasts several hours or days and consists of cholera. You have liquid stools if you have watery diarrhea. This is, for the most part, a sign of a gastrointestinal illness. Water diarrhea can be caused by a variety of microorganisms, including viruses, bacteria, and parasites, some of which are readily treated or do not require treatment.

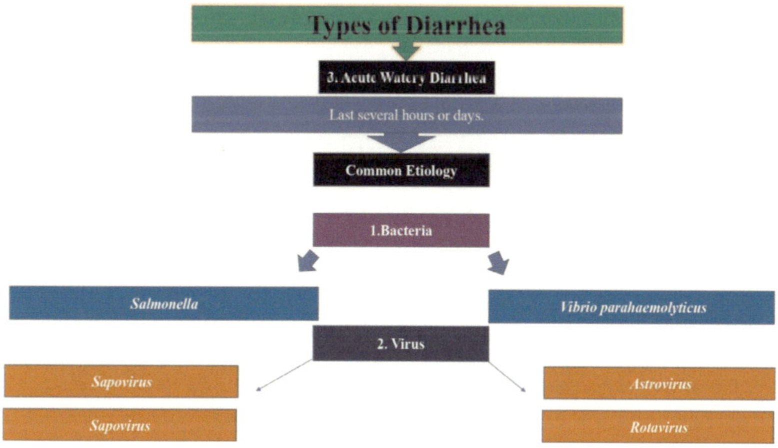

3.2 Acute bloody diarrhea

It is also called dysentery. Acute bloody diarrhea is a health emergency that should be treated quickly. Its cause is usually significant and actionable usually known. Acute bloody diarrhea as a standalone scientific presentation, on the other hand, has received little scientific attention in recent decades. Despite the wide range of probable causes for acute bloody diarrhea, infectious considerations are crucial and should always be prioritized in such patients' evaluations. The goal of the history, examination and laboratory tests should be to get a diagnosis as quickly as possible (and, by extension, to implement appropriate therapy). Adroit therapy for children with acute bloody diarrhea requires carefully planned testing and imaging, avoiding unnecessary diagnostic endeavors, and providing supportive care while waiting for a diagnosis.

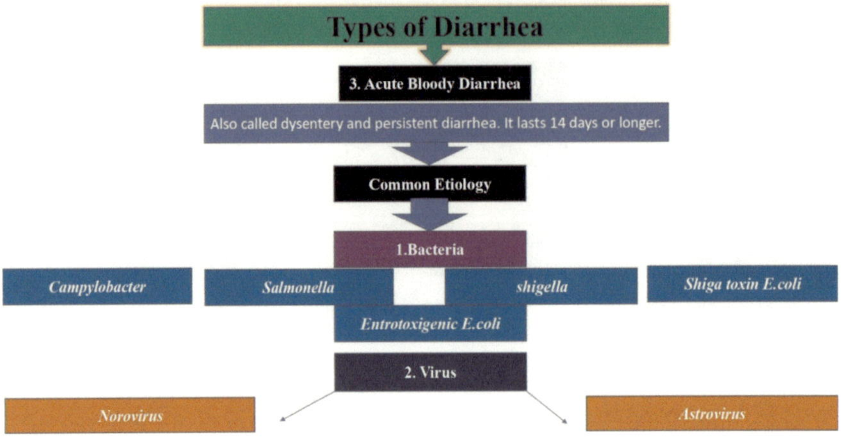

4. Other classification

4.1 Osmatic

A. **Osmatic**

In this type result from the presence of osmotically active poor absorbed solutes in the bowel lumen that

Inhibit normal water and electrolyte absorption.

Causes					
1. ***Bacteria***		**2. Parasite**		**3. Virus**	
Salmonella	*E. coli*	*Cryptosporidium*	*Giardia*	*Norovirus*	*Viral hepatitis*

4.2 Secretory

B. Secretory

It occurs when your intestine cannot properly absorb or secrete electrolyte and fluid.

Causes			
Bacteria- Vibrio cholera	Alcoholism	Medication	Surgery

4.3 Functional

Individuals with functional diarrhea may additionally represent a subgroup of human beings with IBS (irritable bowel syndrome). People with IBS regularly document altered bowel conduct, which includes diarrhea and/or constipation, associated with a stomach ache. Bloating, feeling a pressing want to apply a restroom, straining, or a sense of incomplete evacuation may also occur. Many of those signs arise in individuals with functional diarrhea, however, the absence of abdominal pain distinguishes those humans from those with IBS. People with practical bowel problems no longer exhibit physical or laboratory abnormalities to explain their gastrointestinal (GI) signs. One instance of a purposeful bowel disease is irritable bowel syndrome (IBS), which is envisioned to have an effect on about 10–15% of all adults.

4.4 Acute diarrhea

Acute diarrhea is a syndrome this is regularly now not differentiated clinically by means of a particular etiologic agent. The extensive spectrum of evolution varies from self-confined sickness to demise. Death is particularly because of dehydration and acute diarrhea takes the very best toll among children in low- and middle-earnings nations (LMIC). Acute diarrheal diseases ranked seventh among the reasons of mortality in LMIC in the international disorder burden collection, 2013, with an envisioned 1. Three million deaths (2 Four %).1 Most of those deaths arise in kids under the age of 5 years in LMIC and diarrhea stays among the top 5 causes of all deaths among children more youthful than age 5 years, as tabulated in 2013 [11–20].

5. Causes

5.1 Infective

5.1.1 Bacteria

Which infected the food or water for instance salmonella (salmonella is a group of microorganisms that typically motive meals borne infection. An infection with the aid of the microorganism is known as salmonellosis and you could get it by way of eating infected meals merchandise, which includes uncooked poultry, eggs, beef, and in a few instances fruit. Salmonella has ended up a prime foodborne pathogen throughout the globe, inflicting approximately three.4 million cases and 681,316 annual deaths, with 63.7% of instances occurring in children under 5 years of age [21–22]. There was as a minimum a hundred and fifty non-typhoidal Salmonella serotypes that can purpose gastroenteritis, with *Salmonella Typhimurium* and *Salmonella Enteritidis* being the maximum common serotypes. In terms of control, the recommended empiric parenteral remedy includes cefotaxime or ceftriaxone, while oral therapy consists of amoxicillin, trimethoprim-sulfamethoxazole, or azithromycin. Salmonella isolates have an excessive resistance in the direction of at least one antimicrobial agent, particularly towards clindamycin, oxacillin, penicillin, and vancomycin, for that reason, antibiotic susceptibilities of Salmonella should be determined for the targeted antibiotic therapy and vegetable) shigella and vibrio cholera [23–29].

Viruses also are contributing as the causative agent of diarrhea for example norovirus (Norovirus turned at the beginning known as the Norwalk virus, after the metropolis of Norwalk, OH, wherein the first showed outbreak happened in 1972). This concept is to be the most common purpose of acute gastroenteritis (diarrhea and vomiting contamination) around the sector. It spreads effortlessly through food and drinks and can have a large effect on people's fitness. Norovirus is an emerging cause of acute gastroenteritis, accountable for approximately 17–18% of all acute gastroenteritis cases globally, mainly among advanced international locations [30, 31]. The age organization below one to twelve months vintage has the peak frequency of norovirus infection with extra dangerous factors which consist of intercourse of the [32]. Norovirus is noticed during the year, with the winter and fall (weather seasons) determined to report an improved frequency of illustrations [33, 34]. The finding rate of norovirus cases associates definitely with humidity. Co-contamination with rotavirus [19, 20], astrovirus, and salmonella both may occur in positive cases. Norovirus infections are discovered to reason greater excessive signs of gastroenteritis in children in comparison with rotavirus, especially after the advent of the rotavirus vaccination duration astrovirus.

With an astrovirus-causing acute gastroenteritis' global common prevalence of 11%, the very best prevalence of human astrovirus infections changed inside the organization of youngsters between thirty-seven and forty-eight months old. Human astrovirus contamination particularly takes place for the duration of the dry season in the African continent; meanwhile, the highest occurrence mentioned inside the tropical areas is regularly during the rainy season and winter season in temperate climate countries. Patients commonly manifested with diarrhea, fever, vomiting, and abdominal pain, and rotavirus (It is an epidemic that causes diarrhea and different intestinal symptoms. It's very contagious and is the maximum common cause of diarrhea in toddlers and young children globally. If you observe rotavirus through a microscope, it has a spherical form. The Latin phrase for wheel is "Rota," and is the reason how the virus got its call.

5.2 Non-infective

1. Medicine along with antibiotics, cancer capsules, and antacids that contain magnesium is also taking part in diarrhea problems.

2. Allergies and intolerances to sure food, celiac disease, or lactose intolerance.

3. Radiation therapy, some cancers, and surgical treatments.

4. Malabsorption of food.

5. DM and alcohol.

5.3 Signs and symptoms of diarrhea

- Abdominal cramps or pain

- Bloating

- Nausea

- Vomiting
- Fever
- Blood in stool
- Mucus inside the stool
- Urgent need to have a bowel movement

5.4 Signs of extreme diarrhea

5.4.1 Dehydration

The most serious sign of diarrhea is the lack of water in the body of the person who is facing this disease. In this stage electrolytes like sodium, potassium bicarbonates are not balanced. Another factor is the water imbalance in the body. Other symptoms are vomiting, frequent urination, sweating, stool, and breathing.

- Severe dehydration (as a minimum two of the following symptoms):
- In this stage unconsciousness
- Pinched eyes
- Difficulty in drinking water
- Another sign is the skin pinch and porous is going lower back very slowly (≥2 seconds)

5.5 Examination

On exam it may be diagnosed with sunken eyes, loss of pores and skin turgor, and irritable.

5.6 Health impact

Diarrhea disorder may additionally have bad impact on both bodily and intellectual development. Early formative years malnutrition as a consequence of any cause reduces physical health and paintings productiveness in adults and diarrhea is number one purpose of adolescence malnutrition. It can purpose electrolyte imbalance, kidney impairment, dehydration, and defective immune system response.

Eco-oral Route

Investigation

After cautious history and examination. We will move for investigations.

5.6.1 Blood test

Specific blood antibody assessments can be ordered to assist clarify diagnoses. These can encompass antibodies for precise parasites, celiac disease antibodies, and yeast antibodies.

- Complete blood Hb and TLC (Total Leucocytes Count)
- Serum electrolytes (K+, Na+, Cl-)
- RFT (Renal Function) Test (Urea and creatinine)

5.6.2 Stool test

Stool test is also preferred for the identification of the causative agents of the disease.
For parasites test (eggs and ova).

5.7 Treatment

Most instances of acute diarrhea clear on their own days without remedy. If you have attempted lifestyle adjustments and domestic remedies for diarrhea without achievement, there these ought to be clinical remedies.

- Emergency Management

If the affected person is dehydrated and mentally irritable.

- Pass IV
- Input and 0utput tracking
- Start IV/fluids as an example R/L (Ringer lactate) N/S (Normal Saline) or hemacil.
- Cover antibiotic cover both for aerobes and anaerobe) i.e. ciprofloxacin and fungal.
- Give belly cowl (Risk)
- Once the patient is solid i.e. out of threat, treatment ought to be in keeping with the etiology.
- Antibiotics and anti-parasite tablets for oral use.
- Spasmolytics' i.e. Bascopan, Nospa.
- Give ORS.
- Start ingesting tender meals or liquid weight loss plan e.g., fruit, juice, and so forth.
- If there may be chronic diarrhea, then remedy is according to motive e.g. in IBS we must discover both it is diarrhea dominant, constipation dominant or ache or in celiac ailment e.g., treatment might be according to reason.

5.8 Prevention of diarrhea water

- Through safe water

Most deaths related to diarrhea are due to pathogens received as a result of unsafe consuming water, poor sanitary conditions, and shortage of hygiene. Washing fingers with soap and water get rid of the bacteria, viruses, and parasites that cause ailment. Programmed and activities encouraging humans to clean their hands have been evolved to be used in groups and faculties, consisting of hygiene education, posters, leaflets, comedian books, songs, and drama.

- Adequate sanitation
- Hygiene protection
- Hand washing
- Exclusive breastfeeding for the first six months of existence.
- Food hygiene
- Health schooling about how infections spread.
- Vaccination of Rotavirus

6. Conclusions

Higher cases of diarrhea are seen in developing countries. Diarrheal is the 2nd leading death of children under the age of 5 years old. There are different types of diarrhea that cause number of death every year. Patients of diarrhea are increasing day by day and also increase the causative agents of this disease. First of all, find out the root cause of the diarrhea and a different diagnosis is necessary for the treatment of this disease. Due to the innovation and latest research scientists are able to find out the causes of the disease and at last best management proper sanitation and treatment is the best way of handling this disease.

Acknowledgements

First of all, I am very thankful to The **Almighty Allah** who is the greatest creator of the universe. He blessed and inspired me to complete my research work satisfactorily. I also pay my gratitude with heart and soul to the Holy Prophet (P.B.UH) and his beloved and Holy Family. I offered my heartiest gratitude to my most respected, gracious, highly learned, and reverend research Supervisor **Dr. Muhammad Asrar Choudhary** Assistant Professor Department of Zoology for his consolidated and inspiring guidance.

Thanks

I am really thankful to my group fellows **Zeeshan Yousif, Usama Saleem,** and **Muhammad Faisal** for their love, care, and sincere fellowship. I am really thankful to my Mother Balqees **Anwar, my aunt Khalida akther, and brother Zeeshan Javed w**hose hands always raised for my wellbeing.

May Allah bless all these bright minds with long, happy, and peaceful lives including me (Ameen).

Author details

Zeeshan Javed*, Muhammad Asrar, Bilal Rasool, Rabia Batool,
Muhammad Asad Mangat, Usama Saleem, Muhammad Imran and Amna Batool
Department of Zoology, Government College University, Faisalabad, Pakistan

*Address all correspondence to: zeeshichaudhary7@yahoo.com

References

[1] GBD 2016 Diarrhoeal Disease Collaborators. Estimates of the global, regional, and national morbidity, mortality, and aetiologies of diarrhoea in 195 countries: A systematic analysis for the Global Burden of Disease Study 2016. The Lancet Infectious Diseases. 2018;**18**: 1211-1228

[2] GBD 2017 Diarrhoeal Disease Collaborators. Global, regional, and national age sex-specific mortality for 282 causes of death in 195 countries and territories, 1980–2017: A systematic analysis for the Global Burden of Disease Study 2017. Lancet. 2018;**392**:1736-1788

[3] GBD 2017 Disease and Injury Incidence and Prevalence Collaborators. Global, regional, and national incidence, prevalence, and years lived with disability for 354 diseases and injuries for 195 countries and territories, 1990–2017: A systematic analysis for the Global Burden of Disease Study 2017. Lancet. 2018;**392**:1789-1858

[4] Balasubramanian R, Im J, Lee J-S, Jeon HJ, Mogeni OD, Kim JH, et al. The global burden and epidemiology of invasive non-typhoidal salmonella infections. Human Vaccines & Immunotherapeutics. 2018;**15**:1421-1426

[5] Pui CF, Wong WC, Chai LC, Tunung R, Jyaletchuemi P, Noor Hidayah MS, et al. Salmonella: A foodborne pathogen. International Food Research Journal. 2011;**18**:465-473

[6] Chung N, Wang S-M, Shen C-F, Kuo F-C, Ho T-S, Hsiung CA, et al. Clinical and epidemiological characteristics in hospitalized young children with acute Gastroenteritis in Southern Taiwan: According to Major Pathogens. Journal of Microbiology Immunology and Infection. 2017;**50**:915-922

[7] Wu L, Luo Y, Shi G, Li Z. Antibiotic resistance in nontyphoidal Salmonella infection. Infectious Drug Resist. 2021; **14**:1403-1413

[8] Wen SC, Best E, Nourse C. Non-typhoidal Salmonella infections in children: Review of literature and recommendations for management. Journal of Paediatrics and Child Health. 2017;**53**:936-941

[9] Grivas G, Lagousi T, Mandilara G. Epidemiological data, serovar distribution and antimicrobial resistance patterns of Salmonella Species in Children, Greece 2011–2017: A Retrospective Study. Acta Medica Academica. 2021;**49**:255

[10] Barrett J, Fhogartaigh CN. Bacterial gastroenteritis. Medicine. 2017;**45**: 683-689

[11] Jain P, Chowdhury G, Samajpati S, Basak S, Ganai A, Samanta S, et al. Characterization of non-typhoidal salmonella isolates from children with acute gastroenteritis, Kolkata, India, during 2000–2016. Brazilian Journal of Microbiology. 2020;**51**:613-627

[12] Singh R, Yadav AS, Tripathi V, Singh RP. Antimicrobial resistance profile of Salmonella present in poultry and poultry environment in North India. Food Control. 2013;**33**:545-548

[13] Deng X, Ran L, Wu S, Ke B, He D, Yang X, et al. Laboratory-based surveillance of non-typhoidal Salmonella infections in Guangdong Province, China. Foodborne Pathogens Diseases. 2012;**9**:305-312

[14] Haddadin Z, Batarseh E, Hamdan L, Stewart LS, Piya B, Rahman H, et al. Characteristics of GII.4 Norovirus

Versus Other Genotypes in Sporadic Pediatric Infections in Davidson County, Tennessee, USA. Clinical Infectious Diseases. 2021;**73**:e1525-e1531

[15] Ahmed SM, Hall AJ, Robinson AE, Verhoef L, Premkumar P, Parashar UD, et al. Global prevalence of Norovirus in cases of gastroenteritis: A systematic review and meta-analysis. Lancet Infectious Diseases. 2014;**14**:725-730

[16] Farahmand M, Moghoofei M, Dorost A, Shoja Z, Ghorbani S, Kiani SJ, et al. Global prevalence and genotype distribution of Norovirus infection in children with gastroenteritis: A meta-analysis on 6 Years of Research from 2015 to 2020. Reviews in Medical Virology. 2021;**2021**:e2237

[17] Fang Y, Dong Z, Liu Y, Wang W, Hou M, Wu J, et al. Molecular epidemiology and genetic diversity of norovirus among hospitalized children with acute gastroenteritis in Tianjin, China, 2018–2020. BMC Infectious Diseases. 2021;**21**:682

[18] Cao R-R, Ma X-Z, Li W-Y, Wang B-N, Yang Y, Wang H-R, et al. Epidemiology of Norovirus gastroenteritis in hospitalized children under five years old in Western China, 2015–2019. Journal of Microbiology and Immunology Infection. 2021;**54**:918-925

[19] Mikounou Louya V, Nguekeng Tsague B, Ntoumi F, Vouvoungui C, Kobawila SC. High prevalence of Norovirus and rotavirus co-infection in children with acute gastroenteritis hospitalised in Brazzaville, Republic of Congo. Tropical Medicine & International Health. 2019;**24**:1427-1433

[20] Li LL, Liu N, Humphries EM, Yu JM, Li S, Lindsay BR, et al. Aetiology of diarrhoeal disease and evaluation of viral–bacterial coinfection in children under 5 years old in China: A Matched Case–Control Study. Clinical Microbiology Infections. 2016;**22**:381

[21] Rönnelid Y, Bonkoungou IJO, Ouedraogo N, Barro N, Svensson L, Nordgren J. Norovirus and Rotavirus in children hospitalised with diarrhoea after Rotavirus vaccine introduction in Burkina Faso. Epidemiological Infections. 2020;**148**:e245

[22] Arowolo KO, Ayolabi CI, Adeleye IA, Lapinski B, Santos JS, Raboni SM. Molecular epidemiology of Astrovirus in children with gastroenteritis in Southwestern Nigeria. Archives of Virology. 2020;**165**: 2461-2469

[23] Lu L, Zhong H, Xu M, Su L, Cao L, Jia R, et al. Molecular and epidemiological characterization of human Adenovirus and classic human Astrovirus in children with acute diarrhea in Shanghai, 2017–2018. BMC Infectious Diseases. 2021;**21**:713

[24] Mozhgani SHR, Samarbafzadeh AR, Makvandi M, Shamsizadeh A, Parsanahad M, Jalilian SH. Relative frequency of Astrovirus in children suffering from gastroenteritis referred to Aboozar Hospital, Ahvaz. Jundishapur Journal of Microbiology. 2011;**4**:67-70

[25] American Gastroenterological Association. Medical position statement: Guidelines for the evaluation and management of chronic diarrhea. Gastroenterology. 1999;**116**:1461-1463

[26] Camilleri M. Chronic diarrhea: A review on pathophysiology and management for the clinical gastroenterologist. Clinical Gastroenterological Hepatology. 2004;**2**: 198-206; Deepak P, Ehrenpreis D. Diarrhea. Dis.-Mon. 2011, 57, 490–510

[27] Diarrhoea: Why Children Are Still Dying and What Can Be Done, 2009. The United Nations Children's Fund (UNICEF)/World Health Organization (WHO)

[28] DuPont HL. Bacterial diarrhea. The New England Journal of Medicine. 2009; **361**:1560-1569

[29] Fine KD, Schiller LR. AGA technical review on the evaluation and management of chronic diarrhea. Gastroenterology. 1999;**116**(6): 1464-1486

[30] Lewis SJ, Heaton KW. Stool form scale as a useful guide to intestinal transit time. Scandinavian Journal of Gastroenterology. 1997;**32**(9):920-924

[31] Pawlowski SW, Warren CA, Richard Guerrante R. Diagnosis and treatment of acute or persistent diarrhea. Gastroenterology. 2009;**136**(6): 1874-1886

[32] Thiagarajah JR, Verkman AS. Water transport in the gastrointestinal tract. In: Johnson LR, editor. Physiology of the Gastrointestinal Tract. fourth ed. 2006

[33] UNICEF. Improved Formula for Oral Rehydration Salts to Save Children's Lives. 2006. Available from: http://www.unicef.org/media/media_31825.html

[34] Oral rehydration salts. Available from: http://www.who.int/medicines/publications/pharmacopoeia/Oralrehydrationsalts.pdf